For Ava
It is all for you.
Just you look and see
what I can do!

In the Shade

of

Ava's Tree

Surviving HELLP, Stillbirth, and Rebirth

MELISSA KRAWECKI

Praeclarus Press, LLC

www.PraeclarusPress.com

Praeclarus Press, LLC
2504 Sweetgum Lane
Amarillo, Texas 79124 USA
806-367-9950
www.PraeclarusPress.com

DISCLAIMER
The information contained in this publication is advisory only and is not intended to replace sound clinical judgment or individualized patient care. The author disclaims all warranties, whether expressed or implied, including any warranty as the quality, accuracy, safety, or suitability of this information for any particular purpose.

ISBN: 978-1-939807-40-3

Cover Design: Name Ken Tackett
Back Cover Photo: HRM photography
Copy Editing: Chris Tackett
Acquisition & Development: Kathleen Kendall-Tackett
Layout & Design: Cornelia Georgiana Murariu
Operations: Scott Sherwood

Table of Contents

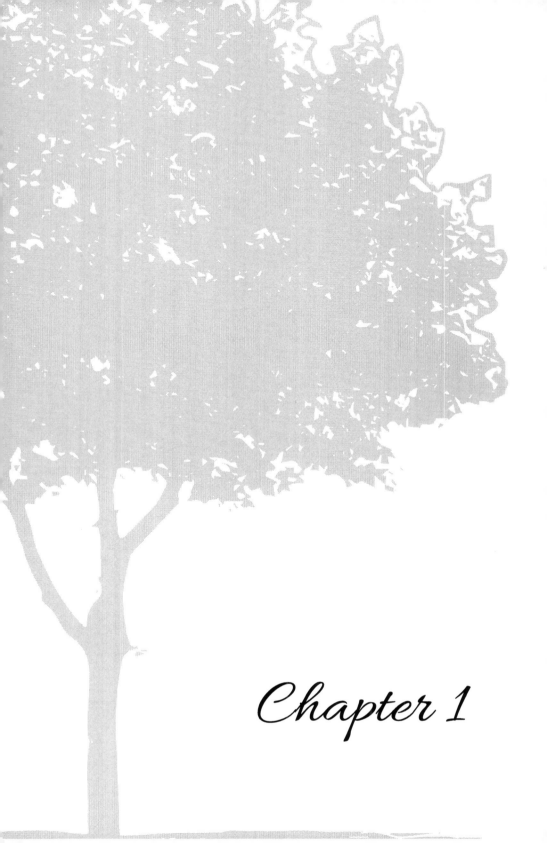

Chapter 1

Ignorance is Bliss

Our story is both naive and ignorant. I think back now, and I see the rose-colored glasses that we viewed the world through. The ones that said every baby lives and bad things happen to bad people.

Boy, were we wrong!

I met my husband in the eighth grade. He was the boy at the back of the bus with the faded Levi's jeans and a flop of dark-brown hair across his forehead. He had the biggest blue eyes I had ever seen, and the kindest soul to match them. Never a show boater, Matthew was the constant in my turbulent and achingly normal teenage experience. He was always there, waiting quietly in the background—probably for me to get a clue that he was there at all. And I finally did, at the tender age of 21. I am not the most astute sometimes, but when I did realize he was there waiting for me, our life together flowed easily. That's what happens when you marry your best friend. You become engaged less than a year later, and it is all rainbows, lollipops, and sunshine from there.

Except when your firstborn dies while still inside you, and your life is nearly taken by a disorder you cannot pronounce, and a nightmare becomes reality.

Matthew and I lived a quiet life those first few years of marriage. We bought a little house and did what every couple that really wants a baby does—we bought a dog. Charlie, the long-eared beagle, was my consummate companion, along with Simon, the oversized Maine Coon cat. Matthew travelled at lot for work, and was often in the United States and Europe. I spent my time working in Social Services and dabbled in home renovations. Who am I kidding? Both of us more than dabbled. We renovated every square inch of our derelict starter home. It wasn't pretty, but it was ours. A 1970s bungalow with all the stylized, vomit accoutrement that you could ever imagine. Orange, paper-thin wool carpet on the basement stairs, fire-engine red shag in the bedroom, and thin, tired wood baseboards that put the shining glory on its dated wonder. We worked at it room by room, and finally, in the summer of 2010, we did our biggest renovation to date: tearing apart the entire basement to turn it into a living room and playroom.

Because I was pregnant. Or rather, we wanted me to be quite shortly. And shortly, in our case, is all it took.

During the renovation, the main floor of our home had two floors worth of belongings crammed into it. Matthew travelled for the majority of the renovation, while Charlie, Simon, and I were all crammed onto the main floor of the bungalow as the contractors were ripping apart and rebuilding downstairs. Our life was covered in drywall dust, in chaos, and with an end goal in mind to get the basement completed so it could be the perfect recreation and playroom. It would be a cozy spot for three to curl up in front of the fire, with a wee one snuggled in our arms.

Matt was only home for one week in June 2010, and that was all it took for me to become pregnant. We had decided a few months before that we wanted to start "trying" in the summer. We had no clue how long it would take us to become pregnant, and I was convinced it was going to take us years. I kept going over the statistics and thinking, we could easily not be able to have kids, if we are going to do this, we need to act soon. I had this little voice in the back of my head that said I would "not have kids." If I only knew just how accurate that little voice was. We jokingly decided to "pull the goalie" in June of 2010, and left it up to whoever decides these things to see what would happen next.

On July 2nd, I got up that morning, excited. Matthew would be home after two long weeks away, and I was lonely. I missed him, and however nice a bedmate Charlie was, I wanted Matt back to be with me. Crammed into the tiny half of the house, I got up that morning and walked around stacked furniture as I made my breakfast. I turned on the TV, which was covering the G8 summit in Toronto, Canada. It blared away about massive protests expected that day, showing B-roll footage of environmentalists, activists, and thugs throwing rocks at police. Great, I thought, just the world to bring a baby into.

That day, I went about my business. It was a Saturday, and coincidentally, Matthew's 27th birthday. I wanted to pick up his gift and do a little fun shopping to prepare for him coming home around 7 that night. I had recently lost a bunch of weight, and thought it would be time to see if I finally fit into my goal size 8s I had been eyeing at the store. Sure enough, I did! I bought a pair on the spot, the little nagging voice in the back of my head saying, "hopefully, with a baby, they will not fit for long." Just to be sure, I couldn't help but pick up a pregnancy test on the way home. We had been trying for one month. My period was due soon, so it couldn't hurt, right?

I had taken a pregnancy test before wishing a different outcome. Not hundreds of times before or anything, but the procedure was not exactly new to me. This was, however, the first time I remember hoping, wishing, and let me be honest, a little terrified as to the outcome of those two lines. And they showed up quickly! As soon as I peed on the stick, there they were, staring up at me. Those two pink lines.

I set the test on the counter and stared.

Oh, my God.

Yup. That is a positive. I looked in the mirror, shocked and dismayed. Did I really just find out I was pregnant on Matt's birthday? As he is thousands of feet in the air, hurtling in a tin can, and I am unable to reach him, and I am pregnant? What on earth was I thinking, taking the test now? My hands went to my belly and I stood is dismay. Pregnant. I am pregnant. My eyes, wide and shocked, stared back at me. Excitement, the type that causes your hands to shake and for a burst of energy to run down your spine filled me completely. I am pregnant! I am pregnant!

The rest of the afternoon was a blur. I set the test on the living room table and walked around with my skinny jeans on, unable to take my eyes and thoughts off of it. We were going to be parents. That was quick! Really quick! Are we ready? How will Matt react?

My mind spun until I could barely sit still. The G8 was winding up to a fury on the TV in the background, protesters demonstrating and turning the downtown streets of Toronto into a warzone, and my Matthew would be flying in there tonight. I turned off the television and curled up with a labor-and-delivery book my sister had given me. After all, I would need it soon.

I know women think of all sorts of crazy and romantic ways to tell their husbands that they are expecting, but I have never been one of those women. Matt and I are very no-nonsense. Not to say we haven't had our share of idyllic romanticism in our day. I just did not feel the need for an over-the-top gesture about a topic I could barely get my head wrapped around. I needed him to know so we could begin the journey together. He was my partner, my best friend, and I needed him on the ground and in one piece so we could both be as shocked and bewildered as I was in that moment.

I took the messenger bag I had gotten him for his birthday and placed the pregnancy test inside. I positioned it so that when he opened it, the test would be the first thing he sees. Also knowing that, being a guy, he may not even know what he was looking at, so I made sure the two positive lines were clearly visible. I do not think Matt had ever seen a pregnancy test, aside from the commercials where the ladies spoke in creepy soft tones, sport non-judgemental faces, and talk about "being sure."

Seeing him that night as he stumbled, thoroughly exhausted and jetlagged, in the door was such a relief. I threw my arms around his neck and buried my head into his chest. We were so used to his crazy travel schedule, but all the sudden things felt different. There was another little person that needed him as much as I did, and he did not even know it yet. I suddenly needed him much closer than ever before.

When the time came for him to open his birthday gift that night, I was on pins and needles. He liked the bag, and was ooing and awing, making all the appropriate, "yes, Melissa, I do like the gift" noises I had taught him to make. He opened up the flap of the bag and was suddenly frozen. He stared hard at those two little lines and looked up at me.

"Are you? Are we?" he asked.

"Apparently!" as I pointed to the two little lines.

I remember hugging and staring at the test together in quiet reflection. No movie-star-couch jumping or grand gestures of emotion. No pregnancy test tied to the dog's collar to greet him or a pink-and-blue cupcake surprise. Just he and I, me on his lap, held close. It was perfect.

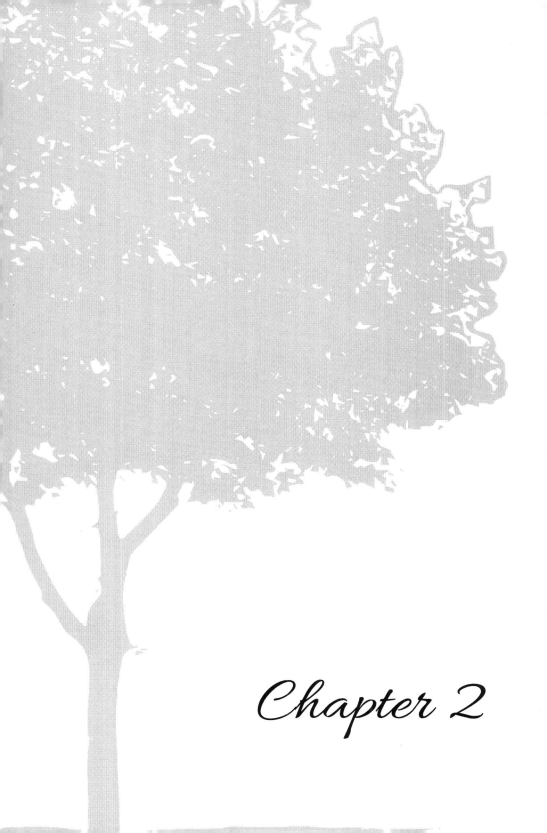

Chapter 2

Our Family of Three

It is a very strange request we put on women to not share their pregnancies. Doctors encourage new moms not to tell anyone for fear of something going wrong, and it is very isolating. You walk around with this loud bell going off in your head: I AM PREGNANT! It is in every squeak of your shoes.

Squeak! I am pregnant.

Squeak! Squeak! I. Am. Pregnant.

It is as loud as a city bell tower, the only word on your tongue, and the only all-consuming thought in your head. Yet, you cannot tell anyone.

And because I had read all the books a year before, I knew it was extra important not to tell anyone. They all said just that.

I went to work the next week, back to the world's tiniest cubicle at my City Hall job. I worked in Social Services as a case manager, and had a very large caseload. I was a contract worker and had no job security whatsoever. I was desperate to be in a full-time, permanent position. I loved my coworkers, my job, and my life working there. I had it in my mind that this would be the perfect job to come back to after taking maternity leave. It meant the convenience of working with set hours to pick up and drop off the baby at daycare. I thought I had struck gold. It was a three-minute drive from home: demanding, challenging, and incredibly high stress. And even with all that, I never felt like I belonged.

Being on the outside as a contract worker, I was always jockeying for a position with the other contract workers for the measly pickings of positions that would come open, perhaps once a year. When I found out I was pregnant, my contract was only confirmed for three more months. Three more months, and if they found out I was pregnant, I knew my contention for a permanent position could be dramatically reduced. So now, I really needed to keep this all-consuming secret from coming out.

Hiding the baby wasn't easy. For starters, I felt horrid. By the time I was six weeks pregnant, the nausea was increasing, and the fatigue blinded me. I had a high-energy job. I could not afford to fall behind. So I pushed, and pushed, and pushed myself to perform.

It meant I spent the first trimester increasingly stressed. Running outside to vomit so to not draw attention to myself vomiting in the bathroom stalls, I would come home from work and go straight to bed, sleeping through from 5 p.m. to 7:30 a.m., and do it all again. I had to make my phone calls to my care providers in my car on break and come up with excuses for the appointments I needed to make. I was flat-out exhausted. Exhausted from hiding the pregnancy, and determined to give us the best chance of security by the time the baby arrived. I believed the best chance of us being financially secure was to have a permanent job to come back to. Little did I know how hard I was being on myself and my baby. How unnecessarily stressful the entire notion of keeping it a secret truly was.

With great relief, my contract was extended past my due date when I was 9 weeks pregnant. Although it was not permanent, I knew I had proven myself to be a reliable and good worker. Surely a permanent spot would come open in the next few months. The night I was extended, Matthew and I opened a bottle of sparklingly non-alcoholic cider and danced in the kitchen. We were going to be just fine. At 11 weeks pregnant, I announced my pregnancy. Being able to finally tell everyone that I was expecting was a huge relief. My coworkers and boss were supportive, and although, the demands of my job only increased with time, a weight began to lift from my shoulders.

Once I was around 11 weeks, the fatigue was less crippling and the nausea was beginning to subside. Filled with joy and unbridled expectation, I set my eyes on preparing for my baby. Of course, I read every book imaginable, believing it would prepare me for the monumental change that was about to happen. My week "12-week officially 2nd trimester" gift to myself was to sign up for prenatal classes. Twelve weeks felt so safe, and I wanted to celebrate that we were in a "safe" zone. I found the best place in my town: Vesta Parenting. Vesta Parenting is a locally run business that provides supports, services, and education for families. They were all about green living and believe that women's bodies were designed to birth.

They were well-resourced in the community. I knew they would be a perfect match for my crunchy, trust-your-body-everything-will-be-fine self.

The day I walked into Vesta, I was greeted with a smile by one of the owners, Shawn; a fiery, henna-dyed redhead, with homemade earrings dangling from her ears. She was loud, open- faced joking with a patron across the counter. When I strolled up and asked her to be enrolled in her January 2011 class, she scoffed at me,

"I don't even have an enrollment sheet for that yet!" It was September. "Aren't you an eager one?"

The store smelled of diaper ointment, and there were wooden baby toys at the cashier till. It was earthy and just the perfect amount of hippy. I was in love. I signed up for my prenatal class and skipped out with joy under my feet. I was going to be a Mama, and I could see myself happily shopping here with my new friends. We would talk about using all-natural oils as salves, and actually use all the reusable bags I had jammed in the corner of my trunk that never made it to the store.

I leapt head first into pregnancy. Before I was even pregnant, I read every pregnancy and labor book I could get my hands on. Taking the lead of my sister before me, she had one child and was expecting her second three months before me. She told me all about my options, and handed over every book and article to consider. After combing through all of the documents, I became convinced of my body's ability to labor, and that less truly would be more in regards to medical intervention. Along that line of thinking, I found myself moved toward midwifery care. Luckily, there happened to be a midwives' office in our town, and I was able to get myself a spot fairly easily.

Going to meet with the midwives was a nerve-wracking experience. A nervous first-time mom, I felt myself rattled by the entire experience of pregnancy. I felt out of my element, a duck out of water, and unsure of what was normal, and what I "should" be feeling. The second I walked into the midwives' office, I felt at ease. Big comfortable sofas, with lovely warm murals all over the walls, welcomed us. The receptionist welcomed us with a broad and lovely smile. Their care was warm and gentle. I eased into them, and knew wholeheartedly that I had made the right choice. I was assigned to a team of midwives, meaning that two of the members of my team would attend my birth. I was assured of their care for the duration of my pregnancy.

On my second appointment with my midwives, I met Laura. Laura was a striking, dark-haired beauty, around my age. With a breezed confidence, she came into the room and introduced herself. She was efficient, soft, and kind in manner, with a phenomenally witty sense of humor. Perhaps what I loved most of all was that she asked something that hardly anyone had:

"Tell me about the baby."

I was gobsmacked. At this point, in the midst of my second trimester, I was just beginning to feel movement and identify with the fact I was pregnant. What I could tell her was:

This baby is gentle and loves the time period from 9 p.m. and 11 p.m., with lots of activity. He or she loves the sound of Matthew's voice, and in bed, we will lie together, and he will talk to the baby. I will feel the baby shift over to get as close as possible to him. Hates chicken, makes me sick instantly. Loves music, is very perceptive, and listens closely to us.

I saw her smile and I could feel it in my toes.

Nesting with the baby felt unending. Our tired, cramped, 1970s, half-renovated home suddenly had every flaw imaginable. Our basement project was moving ahead very slowly. Much too slowly for my pregnant self. The walls and floors were done, and we were in the midst of putting it all back together again. Our friends, Caroline and Logan, came to help paint while I nested, and fussed, and obsessed over each and every detail of our ideal recreation room for the family. I was consumed with finding the perfect leather sofa and love seat for our new space. I wanted to find the perfect wall unit that would store all the toys and kid stuff all neat and tidy. I was in organizational heaven. Spending hours upon hours on Swedish furniture websites designing, redesigning, measuring, and building the perfect living room and playroom for the baby.

I was in second-trimester heaven. One of the greatest joys came from sharing the news of our pregnancy with our family and friends. Our close friends, Jane and Gus, overflowed with joy when we shared the news one day while picnicking in the park. The first of our friends to have kids, their youngest, Anne, was only a few months old, making our babies less than a year apart, more like siblings than cousins. Jane enthusiastically shared maternity clothes, baby items, and advice at will. She was fantastic. We bonded over breastfeeding and onesies, while the boys congratulated each other with cigars and whiskey drinks on the porch. My parents were over the moon at the announcement, dropping their forks mid-dinner when I said the word "pregnant," and throwing their arms around us in joy. Seeing everyone's excitement only fueled our own and drove home the fact we would be bringing home a baby in a few months' time.

Matthew went to Germany again in the fall of 2010, but not before I had us drive two hours to the store to buy all the flat packed new shelving we would need for our living room. And a dining hutch because, of course, babies need a new dining hutch to match the dining table. Matthew slugged and slaved 800 pounds of flat packed furniture into our work minivan, me with burgeoning belly helping where I could. Let's face it, I was a nesting monster. He managed to get all the items inside and stacked neatly, two days before he kissed me and the belly goodbye for what would be his last overseas trip before the baby was born.

As he went out the door, he left strict instructions: I was to leave the boxes alone. In two weeks, he said he would come back and put it all together. It was November 2010, and the baby was not due until March 15th 2011. Just hold your horses.

The holding of horses was not in my plans.

On my second day home alone, after I came home from work, I found myself staring at the dining hutch boxes stacked in the corner of the kitchen. Surely it could not be THAT hard to put together. Surely, I could manage it myself. I did not want to hurt the baby, but figured, what is the worst some Swedish flat-packed furniture could do? Surely I could try.

I started by unpacking the boxes, and figured that if I could unwrap it all and get my bearings as to how to put it together, that would be enough for one night. The first problem was the fact that our kitchen had ceramic floor. The unforgiving, hard, cold, ceramic floor. Kneeling down was uncomfortable on my knees, and bending at the waist was no longer an option. So I laid a towel down on the floor and began to undo all the zip ties, pull at the cardboard and slowly managed to get the first of two boxes unassembled.

By the end of that first night, I had all the parts unpacked, and I had it all sorted into piles according to the pictograph instructions. Not bad! I thought. On the second night, I began to assemble it slowly on the floor. Laying out the pieces, I worked slowly and quietly, happy, cheery music and Charlie the dog to keep me company. Simon would lay on the pieces I was using, naturally, as cats have to be part of the action. It was a fun project. No one knew I was working on it. If Matt knew, he would surely lay an egg in a fit of frustration. Night after night, I puttered away at my hutch, an hour or two until my knees would hurt or my tummy would tighten, and I would know it was time for glass of water and to sit.

On the fifth, night I finally had it all assembled, but there was one problem. The final instruction was to stand it up from its horizontal position on the floor and to set it on its feet to install the glass shelves. I stood there, staring at it, knowing it would be impossible to pick up. So, naturally, I did what most girls do; I called my mom. After pulling the phone away from my ear as she yelled at me through the phone, she agreed to come out after work the next day and to help me set it right.

By the time Matthew came home, I had assembled the dining hutch, rearranged the formal living room, and assembled half the shelves for the new living room downstairs.

In the last few weeks of the pregnancy, I began to feel particularly run down. Having read all the books, I knew that fatigue could increase again in the third trimester, and in so, found myself returning to the old behaviors I had as habit those first few weeks of pregnancy; going to bed right after dinner and dragging myself through the day.

Somehow, it was more than that. I was beginning to feel generally unwell. No one thing would jump out at me in particular, just unwell. I would count the hours to get through the day at work and would often only feel relief when resting. It was unending. At 30 weeks pregnant, it seemed like 40 or even 42 weeks was a lifetime away. I was beginning to slip up at work. I was losing my edge, and I knew I was not going to be able to keep up this pace much longer, and I was scared for my job. Scared about being seen as weak or unable to handle things. At my 30-week checkup with my midwives, I met with someone I do not normally see. She was filling in for my usual midwife and was not on my team. I approached the topic of my fatigue and generally feeling unwell, and immediately, I was cut off.

"Mother's always think they cannot work," she said. "I see women all the time that come in the second they are expecting and want sick leave. Yes, pregnancy is hard but it is manageable."

Immediately dismissed. Immediately diminished. I felt shame rise through my body. The color rose in my cheeks, and I found myself agreeing with her, yes, pregnancy is hard. Yes. It is manageable.

I walked out of the appointment, and decided I just needed to try harder. If I just tried harder, I wouldn't feel so bad. If I just tried harder, I could be better at this. I could just think myself into feeling better.

Three weeks later, I was almost 34 weeks pregnant and returning back to my midwives for a follow-up. This time, another new face met with me. Her kind heart, warm smile, and soft English accent were instantly welcoming. Although, she wasn't Laura, I felt a bond there instantly. I felt myself compelled to tell her what every fiber of my soul was screaming; I am not well.

"I just don't feel well," I said, half looking at the floor, waiting to be told a snide "welcome to motherhood" one liner.

"Oh?" I looked up and saw her blue eyes trained on me. Tears caught in my throat and I sputtered,

I just don't feel well. I am tired. Really tired. I have this job and I don't want to lose it. I want to be a good employee, but I know I am slipping up. I go home, make dinner, and fall into bed. I feel like crap. All the time—not sometimes. All the time. I cannot keep doing this.

"Well, that isn't good, my dear," she said. Her tone was calm and compassionate. "Let us see if we have tested your levels." She flicked through my chart and immediately saw we had not tested my iron levels. She quietly and calmly took my blood sample, and said she would send it to the lab. "Now tell me about your work."

With her bright eyes burrowing into mine, it all came out; "I work contract and I really want to be hired on permanent. If I can just manage to show them that I am committed to staying there, they may reconsider me when my mat leave is up. I figured I would work as long as I could so that maybe, perhaps, there would be an opening that I could get hired on permanent before I left on leave..." Gigantic, tired tears rolled down my cheeks.

Suddenly, her hand was on mine in my lap. "Being pregnant is hard. You have to listen to your baby. If you are ready to be done work, then you are ready. There is no shame in that."

"But I am only 34 weeks pregnant!" I felt shame rise through my body and find its way into my cheeks. Shouldn't I be able to do it all?

"So you are 34 weeks pregnant! Listen to your baby. Your baby is telling you it is time to just be, Mama. It isn't about pride or anything else. It is about what your baby needs."

It was February 2, 2011, and I knew it was time to stop work. In that sentence, I was given the permission to take care of me. As I trudged down the two flights of stairs to the parking lot, I felt resolved for the first time in weeks. Pulling in the driveway, it was pitch black outside, and I could see Matt puttering in the kitchen. I sat in the driveway and watched him a moment. This would be my focus now: home. Such relief washed over me.

"Hey, hot stuff. How was the appointment?" Matt's smile greeted me in the door as I waddled in.

"Hey. Well, I think I need to go off work."

He looked up from the dishwasher; "Okay. Then that is what we do." That was it. No further discussion needed. I could see he was a bit thrown by the notion, but didn't question it.

The next morning, I got up and went into work, and gave my notice for a week later. I did not know what would happen with my job security, or lack thereof, but I knew it was time. Still tired, still feeling ill, I thought I could manage through seven more days of work.

The baby shower and open house were fast approaching. Set for February 5, 2011, it was the goal for the many weeks of preparation we had completed on the house. Matthew had finished painting and installing every last piece of trim in the house. The basement renovation was completed, the nursery prepped, even the caterer was booked, so I would not have to cook. Over 30 people had RSVP'd yes, which shocked us. Furthermore, how would we fit them all in our tiny house? We did not even care. This was about our baby and it would be fine... That is, as long as all of them did not show up all at once. Even my brother and his family were coming down for the event. Chris is the consummate older brother, the protector, and the one who picks on you the worst of all. My pet name for him is hardly kind on the outset: Jackass. But Christopher is. He is heart and soul, brash and ruthless. Driven and high achieving to his core, Christopher is at the top of his game in all that he works towards. Living some six hours away by car, in February, driving through the Snow Belt, I was well aware of what he was doing to come to our baby shower.

And I was grateful.

On the day before the baby shower, I was finishing up my work week. Anxious to get out of there, I went to the flower shop to pick up some flowers to make decorations for the party. I wanted both of the bathrooms and the living room to have beautiful flowers to be welcoming. I had seen all my friends do it at their big events, and this was big. This was our home's debut! All the renovations, all the work, with all our family and friends there! This was not only our first child's baby shower, but also a coming out of sorts for our little house and all we had done.

The morning of the shower, I woke up and stood up beside the bed. Underneath my right breast, my ribs ached. Odd, I thought. I stretched over my head from side to side and attempted to get my lungs some room. The baby's head was really low and feet were up in my ribs. Breathing was beginning to be difficult. Stretching did not help it. I waddled around the house, feeling rather horrid and generally unwell. I would find myself, from time to time, putting my hand over the ribs on my right side. I felt as if I needed to hold the area. With the shower slated to begin at 2 p.m., our house was a flurry from early on. The flowers were perfectly arranged—beautiful, white, and fragrant—that cheerily went against the dark gloom of February outside. The snow was coming down in feet that day, constant and unabiding. In the tiny bungalow, it felt warm and inviting out of the snowfall.

As the caterer arrived, it began to snow. Everything was set up, and before I knew it, the house was packed with aunts, uncles, friends, and loved ones. Feeling as miserable as I was, I attempted to host as much as I could, but often found myself just wanting to sit and rest. I nibbled on food a little, but was not very hungry. My nerves were up. This long-anticipated day was palpable with joy. I sat back and watched my loved one finally together, all celebrating our baby.

At one point, I sat down with the women in my family and I mentioned the odd pain I was having, this rib pain.

"Oh, it is just because the baby is kicking you," my one aunt said.

"Just you wait until those legs get stronger! Then you will be really sore." The cackling of laughter did little to comfort me. It was still there, and its constant nature was beginning to worry me.

My sister, Kath, brought her sweet boy, Leo, with her. At just under 6 weeks old, this was a coming out of sorts for him too. I curled up on the sofa with Chris and Kath as we all held Leo together, and it was the most complete I remember feeling in years. All of us together, celebrating new life. It would be the last time I ever remember feeling complete, probably for the rest of my life.

"Do you have names yet?" Chris asked.

"We have a couple, but are struggling with girl names. Any suggestions?"

"If I had a girl, I like Emma. And Ava."

Ava is a family name; my great grandmother's name is Ava. Emma is beautiful as well, but Ava. I instantly added that to the top of the list.

As the open house wore down, and guests unburied themselves from the massive snowfall that kept coming down all day long, I began to take stock of the damage. Kath and sister-in-law, Kim, graciously cleaned up the house and put everything away before leaving. I waddled down to put on my PJ's, and Matt and I thought we may grab a few leftovers for a late supper after all the commotion.

As I sat down with my plate of finger foods and cold veggies, I put my feet up on the ottoman. I looked down at my feet and they were unrecognizable! My feet and ankles were incredibly swollen.

"Matt! Come here!" I cried out, horrified. "Look at my feet! This is unreal!"

"Whoa!" he said, "Look at them! Is that normal?"

"Well, some women's feet swell later in pregnancy. And it is just my feet and ankles, so I guess so."

"That doesn't look like it should be normal. You rest."

He went upstairs to grab his food and brought down a heat pack for my aching back and ribs. I sat there and nibbled, the heat not even registering to help the constant pain in my ribs.

The next morning, I woke up feeling just as horrid as the day before. Instead. now the pain was between my shoulder blades. The swelling in my feet and ankles was now in my legs and I felt like a puffer fish. I knew right away I would need to rest that day. I spent most of the day on the sofa, with my heat pack on my back. There were times when I felt like maybe it was helping, and other times when I knew it wasn't. It did not make sense to me. I dosed and watched movies. Around 3 p.m., I started to get bored, so I convinced Matthew to help me put together the brand new playpen we had received as a shower gift. I read the instructions and he put it all together. It was every dream I ever had about becoming a parent with him. When it was all set up, we grabbed the mobile and attached it to it. I turned it on and we stood there for a moment, listening to the "Twinkle, Twinkle

Little Star" nursery rhyme. Matt had his arm around my shoulders, and I could just picture bringing this person home and using this playpen and changing table in the basement, cozied up by the fire for the winter together.

But I felt horrid. I was sore, swollen, puffy, and generally bad.

The next morning, I felt no better. I was surprised. I had rested the entire day before and normally, that helped me. I thought about not going into work, but I knew my bosses were aware of my baby shower on the weekend and this was my last week. It would not look good if I did not show up to work, and I so badly wanted to belong there. I couldn't leave them in a lurch. If resting did not help it, then what would staying home do?

Going out the door that day to work, I turned to Matthew and promised if I felt worse, I would come home and call the midwife. He bent down to kiss me and I could smell his aftershave.

"I think it is a boy," I said sweetly.

"Oh? You have always said it is a girl," he questioned.

"I know, but I feel like a surprise is coming."

If I only knew.

Getting into work, I felt very restless. I heated up my heat pack and laid low in my tiny cubicle. Around 9 a.m., I decided I would contact the midwives and see what they said. Going out into the hallway when they returned my call, we chatted.

"Hey, guys. I am sorry to bother you. I have been having a weird pain and I do not know what to think of it."

"Can you describe the pain for me?"

"It is beneath my left shoulder blade and constant. I think the heat is helping, but I can't really tell. It started this weekend."

"Are you seeing any spots? Headache?"

"I have a touch of a headache. I took an acetaminophen and that seems to be helping."

There was a long pause.

"Well, being that the acetaminophen is helping and your blood work came back okay from this week ... maybe the baby is just pushing up on your ribs and causing some pain. Could just be muscular. If your pain worsens, or if you start to have a bad headache, seeing spots, then it is time to call us and get into the emergency room. Okay?"

Her request seemed reasonable. I nodded and thanked her. I hung up and called my massage therapist and booked in for a 5 o'clock appointment. Perhaps a massage could help me feel more comfortable.

I just could not get this unsettled feeling that there was something more going on. I went through the day, motion by motion.

At 3 p.m., I got a sudden feeling to stand up, and my feet were making their way to my boss' office. Much like that feeling where you feel like you may throw up, and you find yourself making your way to the bathroom. This was akin. I waited outside her office for 10 full minutes as she was on the phone, knowing I needed to go home. Now.

Suddenly, a feeling washed over me. A translucent, sparkling sensation. I felt out of my body a moment, and I heard a loud, ringing bell. A strong urge came over me: "GO HOME!" it said. I walked into a nearby office and told the staff there to tell our boss I had to go.

I walked as fast as I could to my desk. I didn't even pick up my glasses or lunch bag. I grabbed my coat and walked as fast as I could to my car.

"Hang on, baby," I pleaded. "I do not know what is wrong. But I will figure it out." My hand was on my hard belly as I walked faster and faster.

It was 3:15 p.m. on February 7, 2011, and I knew something big was coming.

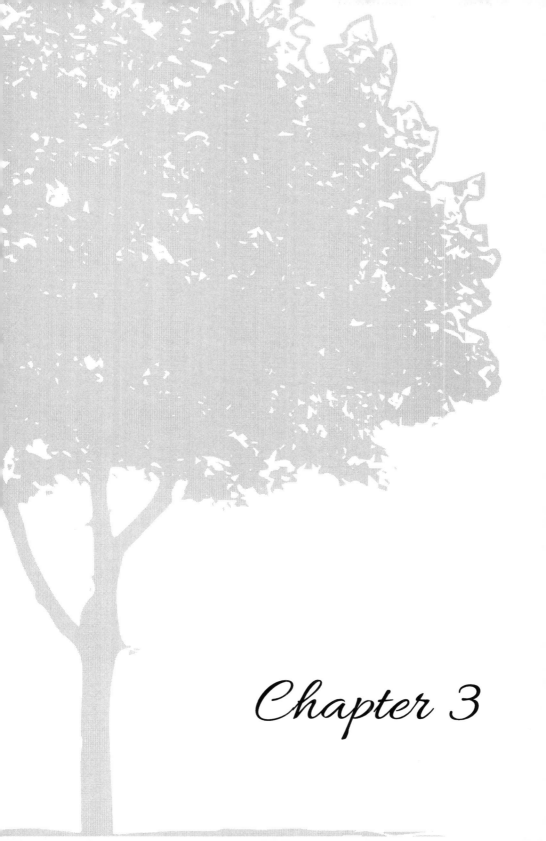

Chapter 3

HELLP Me

At 6:00 that night, after many conversations with my midwives by phone, I decided the pain was concerning, and it was time to go to the emergency room. By this point, the only position I was comfortable in was laying down. If I stood up straight, I was in crippling, grunting, unimaginable back pain, underneath my left shoulder blade. We got me in the car, and I had to put the car seat all the way back and lie looking at the ceiling. Matt drove as fast as he could.

"It will be okay, babe." I said. "It will. It will."

He was lost in his own world, just trying to drive us there quickly. I stared up at the street lights reflections on the ceiling of the car. "This isn't the drive to the hospital I thought it would be," I thought.

Once parked in the emergency parking lot, Matt came around to help me out of the car and I yelped in pain. So intense. It was burning, constant, crippling pain right underneath my left shoulder blade. It did not make sense. These weren't contractions. It was constant, awful, consuming pain. Bewildered, Matthew crutched me into the hospital, where we stood in line for triage.

After waiting 10 minutes to see a nurse, they directed me to sit in the triage chair.

"What are you doing here?" she asked, staring at my belly.

"I am in pain. So much pain. Underneath my shoulder blades. My midwife said to come to emergency. Something is wrong."

The nurse quietly took my vitals and told me to transfer to a nearby wheelchair.

"You do not belong here. You are pregnant. I will have someone take you to the Obsetrical floor."

I told Matt to call our midwife, Laura, and tell her where we are. They pushed me upstairs in the wheelchair to the Obstetrical floor. Upon arriving, we were met by another nurse, who asked us the very same question: "What are you doing here?"

"Please," I begged, "Help me. I am in so much pain, underneath my shoulder blade. I can barely breathe."

"Any contractions?"

"No."

"Any fluid loss?"

"No. My midwife, Laura, told me to come in. She is meeting us here. Please."

"Okay. Lay down on this bed and we will check on the baby. Here, put this on," handing me a hospital gown, "and we will come back in and monitor the baby."

Getting out of the wheelchair was excruciating. Matthew walked me over to the bathroom. I stood in the bathroom, so weak, I couldn't even turn the light on. Leaving the door open so Matt could help me, I undressed. I remember my bra falling to the floor and when I bent down to pick it up, I cried out in pain.

"Leave it, baby, leave it," Matt said. I looked at his eyes and they were so worried.

Oh, this is bad.

Stumbling to the bed, I laid down and took a big breath. On my back, I could breathe and focus. The pain, suddenly, was not so bad. Lying down there was relief, a pressure off. I began to look around the room and realized my surroundings for the first time. A standard birthing room; I could see the equipment surrounding me for a hospital birth.

"This isn't how I thought this would go," I said, absentmindedly.

Matt's face looked drawn. I could see his agreement.

The nurse came in suddenly and said that she was going to put a monitor on my belly to listen to the baby. I told her again about the pain and she nodded as she strapped the stretchy elastic bands on to my stomach. Glancing at the monitor, she then said, "Yup. Nice and strong," as the sound of the baby's heartbeat filled the room.

Oh, sweet baby, I put my head back and breathed. *There you are, little one.* My own heart was racing and I felt horrid. I was gripped with anxiety and confusion. I took several deep breaths and talked to my wee one. "There you are. Hang on, baby. Mama's going to get this figured out."

Matt was pacing the room. He was on the phone with my parents, telling them what was happening, and telling them to come to the hospital. From there, he called Katie again to update her as to where we were. I laid with my eyes shut, breathing into our baby, when the nurse returned.

"The doctor has reviewed your file and has found that this is not a pregnancy-related concern."

"What does that mean?" Matt asked, his blue eyes fierce.

"The doctor has reviewed your file and has found that this is not a pregnancy-related concern. We are transferring you to the emergency department."

"But we JUST came from there!" Matt's tone was suddenly as fierce as his eyes, and I could barely raise my eyes to him. "You have to help her. Please." His tone was now more conciliatory.

"I am sorry, there is nothing we can do. I will help you get back down to emergency." She motioned towards the wheelchair.

"Don't," Matt snapped. "I will help her." He gently came over and took my arm. "Come on, babe."

Sitting up, I gasped in shrieking pain. "Oh God, Matt!"

"I know, babe. Let's just get to the emergency and we will figure this out."

Matt pushed my chair out of the room and we met up with my midwife, Laura, in the hall. Laura took one look at me and I could see her alarm. Matt explained to her that we were being transferred back to emergency as "this wasn't a pregnancy-related concern."

In the emergency room, we met with my parents, and suddenly, we were united, Matthew, Mom, Laura, and I, in figuring out what on earth was going on with me. I transferred to a hospital bed and was allowed to lay down once again. I took a deep breath, and Laura asked me if I wanted to hear the baby.

"Oh yes, please!"

She raised the Doppler to my belly and a heartbeat came through clearly. All four of us smiled at each other with hope. Okay, the baby is okay. Let's figure out what is wrong with me now.

A new doctor entered the room. Tall, fair-haired, with a young, kind face, Dr. Bishop introduced himself. He looked over my chart and said that we had to find the cause of this pain. He consulted with Laura and asked if he could take some blood work. As well, he stated that he wanted to have me do an x-ray to look and see if there was a clot in my lung.

"Is that safe for the baby?" I asked.

"We can make it safe," he said. He listed off the risks to both of us, but stated that if there was a clot in my lung, that it could be life threatening. I turned to Matt and asked him what he thought.

He worked in x-ray and had a very good understanding of the radiation I was about to experience. "They will protect the baby."

In the meantime, Dr. Bishop said they would start me on a morphine drip to help with the pain.

After blood work, I was asked to transfer to another wheelchair and was sent down to the x-ray department.

"You will need to take off all your jewelery," the nurse advised.

I had on my heart-shaped diamond necklace that Matt had given me for Christmas. I took it off and handed it to Matt. My wedding ring and engagement ring needed to come off too. Begrudgingly, I handed them over. I never take my rings off. Matt promised he would keep them safe.

In the x-ray department, they covered my belly with lead as Matt went to talk to the technician who would be taking the x-rays. A few quick shots and I was back to my emergency room bed, with morphine, and everyone waiting.

The morphine wasn't really doing much for the pain. Ripping, constant, sharp, stabbing pain, right underneath my left shoulder blade. It merely lowered it from a 10 on the pain scale to a 9.5. In and out, the nurses came as we would wait for results. Dr. Bishop returned and states that they did not find any clot in my lung. That he had one other idea as to what this pain may be and said they needed to do one more blood test to be sure. After it was done, and the nurse had left once more, Laura asked if I would like to hear the baby's heart beat again.

I laid back and watched Laura's face as she put the Doppler to my belly. Nothing came through. A long silence followed. Laura repositioned the Doppler once more on my belly, moving it from the top of my belly, downwards towards my left hip. All of the sudden, the familiar, "thump thump thump" came through.

"Oh," Laura said, "the baby must have moved. There it is."

But I had not felt the baby move. Adrenaline ripped through my body. *I had not felt the baby move.* I glanced up at the clock on the wall. It's 9:30 p.m. Why isn't the baby moving? Nine p.m. was always baby party time. Breathing shallow breaths, I looked down at my belly. I could not remember the last time I had felt the baby move.

Oh, God.

Just then, Dr. Bishop came back into the room.

"I have a diagnosis for you," he said. "You have HELLP syndrome."

I glance up at Laura and see her soul sink into her body. *HELLP syndrome? What is that?*

"HELLP syndrome stands for Hemolysis, Elevated Liver Enzymes, Low Platelets. It is a pregnancy-related condition of which the only cure is to deliver the baby. The pain you are feeling is liver pain."

"But I am only 34+6. What about the baby?"

"Because you are less than 36 weeks, we have to transfer you to the nearby Catholic hospital in the next city. They are equipped and have a NICU in case the baby requires extra attention."

"So you want us to go there?" Matt asked.

"Yes. We will be taking your wife by ambulance. You can follow in your car."

Suddenly, it hits me just how grave this is. I glance at Matt and see the same thought going through his mind. By ambulance? Is this that serious? Suddenly, the room was filled with people. Nurses taking out my IVs and the paramedics are wheeling in another bed for me to transfer onto. My family members kiss me goodbye, and Matt and I share a long look.

In the ambulance, I follow the route they are taking as we wind through our small town and into the nearby city. I hear the sirens overhead and feel them brake for intersections and speed up where they can. I had driven between our two towns a thousand times and knew the route well. As I followed their path in my head, I put my hands on my belly and talked to my baby. I begged and pleaded for him or her to live. I said I was doing everything I could, large tears rolling down my face. For the first time, I let myself cry.

"I am so sorry, sweet baby," I pleaded. "I am so sorry. I do not know why Mama's body is broken. Please, baby, please just hang on. Oh, your Daddy can't wait to meet you. I promise you I will do everything I can to make it be okay. Mama will try."

Being wheeled into the Catholic specialty hospital, I was determined. I had just spent the last half an hour promising this baby I was going to fight, and fight I was going to do.

I was greeted by a friendly-faced nurse. She smiled at me and said that they were going to get the doctor who would start the induction. I suddenly remembered I had not completed a birth plan yet. That was supposed to be done in three days.

"I want to breastfeed," I told her. "I know you need to know. Will I be able to?"

"Lots of preemies can breastfeed," she assured me.

The room was busy with nurses coming in and out. I was transferring onto the hospital bed when I saw Matthew arrive. He was standing in the hallway with a clipboard and was answering a barrage of questions from a nurse. He looks tired, I thought. It must be really late.

Matt came to my side, and we waited for the doctor to join us. The nurse was just starting my IV when he came into the room.

"My name is Dr. Dewitt." He made no eye contact with me or my husband. His face downturned into my chart, his cold, standoffish nature immediately set me back. "You have HELLP syndrome. We need to check on the baby's position prior to us beginning induction. We will do an ultrasound of the baby and then start the Pitocin."

He looked up from his chart. "Any questions?"

Both Matt and I shook our heads no.

The ultrasound technician came in. A young girl. Matt was by the head of my bed, helping me with my pillows.

"This will feel a little cold," she said as she sprayed the jelly onto my stomach.

The screen was pointed away from us as she scanned my tummy. She went over and over one spot on my belly repeatedly. She then clicked the screen off, looked down at her feet, and said, "I just need to get the doctor."

I took Matthew's hand. Filled with fear, I gripped his hand hard. This cannot be good, to go and get the Doctor. I look up at Matthew and see his tired eyes. I know what is about to come for us, and I am terrified. I know what this means. Just then, I looked up and saw Dr. Dewitt enter the room. The door was wide open into the hallway as he began to scan my belly. I looked through the doorway and saw my mother standing there, her eyes tired.

Dr. Dewitt suddenly turned the screen around to face us. The baby's profile was on the monitor. "I am sorry," he said, "your child has expired."

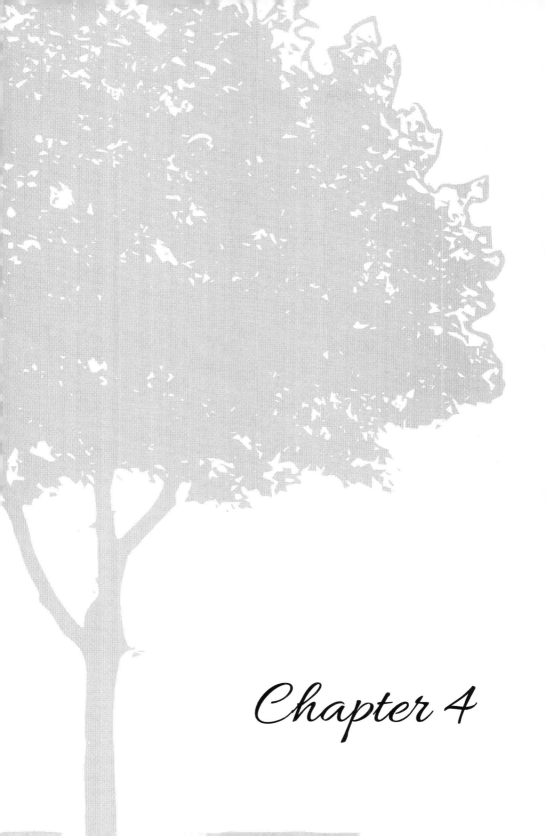

Chapter 4

Expired

Lying on that bed, I stare at the completely still profile of my beautiful child on the monitor.

My Mom had heard it from the hall.

Matthew's hand grips mine hard.

The room spun. I turn my face to his and say, "Oh, God. We killed our baby."

My Mom's face breaks out in pained horror, and we are left in emotional chaos.

I clung to Matthew's shirt and did not cry. We held each other, staring at the ultrasound monitor in complete silence. Dr. Dewitt left us in our silence, my Mom now at my side. The first question I ask is,

"Why? Why, Mama! Why?"

Her eyes fill with tears and she shakes her head no. She has no answer for me. Blinding, horrific heartbreak fills me.

I did not scream. I did not cry. I asked a lot of questions. *Why? How? What is happening? Why didn't you get the baby out in time? Why didn't we know the baby was in distress? How could you let this happen? You said the baby was fine!*

I received no answers. I received pity. I received pained faces that walk into the room and a symbol put on the door to signify a dead baby was within.

I shut off. I went inside to be with my child. I hung onto my child.

I tell her I want to feel nothing. I tell her I want an epidural. I want to be as numb as possible. She nods compassionately and says she will talk to the doctor. The room fills with people. I hear Dr. Dewitt talking to Matthew. I see his lips moving, but have no comprehension of what he is saying. Words do not matter. My baby is dead. *My baby is dead.* The nurses have come and taken out the ultrasound machine, and are beginning to prep the room for my induction.

"Melissa would like an epidural." Matt's words come through clearly in the fog.

"I am sorry," Dr. Dewitt says cooly. "Due to the fact that her platelets are so low with the HELLP syndrome, she cannot have an epidural. We will try and make her comfortable." He turns and walks out of the room.

"I am so sorry, babe," Matt murmurs into my ear. I look up at his eyes and see he is reeling and scared. A mirror image of what I must look like. The room around us is swirling. A nurse is starting an IV drip of magnesium sulphate. I hear her reeling off side-effects, and decide to tune out.

Do what you want with me. I do not matter now.

My midwife Laura comes in, and I see her pained expression from the doorway. I am instantly relieved to see her and grip her hand like an anchor in the storm.

"Why, Laura, why did the baby die? How did this happen? Did we kill the baby?"

Laura's pained light eyes burn into mine. "I do not know. I am so sorry, Melissa. I am so sorry, Melissa," she said. I grip onto her hand and reel. Laura has always told me the truth. How can she not know?

"I am in so much pain, Laura. My back," gasping between breaths, "I can't take much more of this."

"Tell me about the pain," she asked as she had a thousand times before.

"Sharp." Gasp. "Constant." Gasp. "Bad, Laura, bad."

"On a scale of ten?"

"Fifteen! Please!"

"Okay, let me talk to the doctor." With that, she left.

The magnesium sulfate was beginning to take effect and I could feel the room getting even hazier than before. My Dad came in and took my hand as each person had before. From my bed, I could see the doorway was constantly open as people came in and out. Two nurses were assigned to me, and now one sat at the foot of my bed, on constant watch. I tried to make as little eye contact as possible. I was completely overwhelmed and in agony. They had started the Pitocin drip and I had yet to feel a single contraction.

My room was packed with people. It was the middle of the night, my Dad in the corner on a chair, my mother pacing and sitting when possible, and Matthew, stoic at the head of my bed and not moving. We were floating on a sea of chaos. Paper print-out, blood samples, IV drips—and my baby, gone.

Dr. Dewitt returned to the room and stated that they were going to "ripen" my cervix and get the labour progressing. He wanted to insert some gel to ripen it.

It is now 1:00 a.m. I am in horrific, screaming, stabbing pain from my liver. It is rupturing and bleeding out into my abdomen, but no one knows. It is bruising, covering itself in a bruise so deep, it would cover 80 percent of this large organ in my body. No one knows. They remain fixed on delivering "this baby vaginally." They remain fixed on the fact that is best. Dr. Dewitt is not permitting any pain medication other than an ineffective morphine drip, as my liver ruptures, and I begin to contract to deliver my baby into a storm of chaos.

I am so thirsty; I haven't drank anything since 5:00 p.m. the day before. I beg for water. I beg like a dog. They do not allow me a sip for hours. Finally, they allow me to rinse my mouth if I promise never to swallow a morsel. Short-sighted cruelty.

My poor, sweet husband is reeling. He is stunned, as we all are. At every opportunity, I take his hand and tell him I am fighting. I tell him I will survive. I tell him he needs to get me someone who can help me and I will fight. All of my people are completely worn thin. I need someone fresh and willing to fight for me. I ask for Kath, my big sister and second Mama. She is a warrior woman. A force of nature. We now have Kath, Laura, and my parents battling for my life alongside us.

They put in a cervical catheter—unmedicated—to induce labor. It does not work. It is the second worst pain. I scream out in agony and beg them to stop. The pain is horrid, but nothing tops the liver. They put me on Pitocin, I feel a few contractions, but it is a bit like having a foot run over by a car and being concerned with the paper cut on your hand. Inconsequential. I can see by the faces of my family members and husband that they are fighting the doctor to have it be understood that this pain cannot be sustained. That we need to investigate the "upper quadrant" pain further and that action must be taken. It falls on deaf ears. The doctor refuses to listen to us. I am being told to rest, and being poked, prodded, and touched every minute. Can you sleep while someone checks your cervix? Me neither. As if sleep is possible when you are holding your baby in your belly, knowing these moments are the last. When you are told to shift in bed, and you feel the baby's body slump inside you, lifeless. Sickening. I am bitter, enraged, in quiet agony.

I remain in this place for hours, in pain, writhing, and begging for mercy, waiting to dilate, and having no answers, until suddenly, at 7 a.m., shift change occurs.

A new group of what feels like 20 some people to touch, power trip, not listen to me, and tell me what to do. I was less then enthused. That was, until I met my new doctor. His name is Dr. Lopez. He comes over to my bedside and takes my hand. He listens to me with earnestness and his pained concern is evident, even through the hazed cocktail of medications I am swirling in.

"This pain isn't normal. Something is really wrong with me."

Laura, now renewed alongside Kath are in the hall with him explaining, fighting, advocating. He actually listens. Induction continues. However, he starts to run tests to investigate the crippling back pain. It is now mid-morning on February 8, 2011, and the pain increases ever more. I am dilated about 5 centimeters, the contractions are not even noticeable next to the excruciating pain ripping through my right side, my ribs, back, and neck. We do an ultrasound and they see blood in my abdomen. They then order a CT. Now the room is spinning, and every person imaginable is there. My tiny delivery room is packed with people. My ineffective pain medication is stopped and they transfer me to another bed to wheel me to CT. My world is chaos, pain, and confusion. My parents are terrified, and Kath is somehow holding on to everyone with fear in her eyes. I clutch Matt's hand as we are run down to CT. I moan on the table. The pain is increasing as they visualize my liver. They finally know what we have all along. *I am dying.* Part of me wishes I could die alongside my baby, but I will never leave my Matthew.

I am taken back to my room, and I am met with Dr. Lopez and a new face. As I am wheeled into the room, I see a man standing in full motorcycle gear, complete with helmet tucked under his arm. I wipe my eyes in disbelief and wonder,

"Am I hallucinating?"

He begins to speak with authority and introduces himself as Dr. Hernandez. He is soft spoken, powerful, and kind. He tells me they must transfer me to a nearby hospital, where he is the head liver transplant specialist. Dr. Lopez sees my confusion and does not sugar coat it,

"Melissa, you are dying. We must operate to save you."

Dr. McMillan then steps forward and introduces himself. He is a gynecologist and he will deliver the baby by C-section, and at the same time, Dr. Hernandez will access my liver to stop the bleeding. I will have two incisions: one C-section incision and one for the liver. The liver is a large organ and the scar will run across the entire length of my abdomen and down a few inches. Confused, I look up to my family. My mother breaks down in the hall just outside our room. Matthew is in shock. I nod in agreement and take my father's hand and ask him to pray with me. After a quiet prayer, we transferred to a hospital a few blocks away.

As I ride in the ambulance, I begin to pray. I beg for mercy and for absolution. I beg for courage and fight. I know I must stay with Matthew, and now is the moment to dig deeper than ever before. Matthew is with me. Running down the halls of the new hospital, we are met by a team of surgeons. They say Matthew has to stay here and that I must go. I take his hand in mine, and promise him I will fight. I will never leave him. I tell him I love him and hold onto us for me. We cry as we separated.

Wheeling me into the OR, they immediately transfer me onto the operating table. The room is filled with people, at least 20 faces, half of whom are franticly attempting to prep for surgery. I notice they are all fully gowned, with their scrubs tucked into rubber boots up to their knees. Like they are about to go wading, in what? My blood?

The morphine drip has entirely worn off and I am grunting in pain.

"Please! Please! Just put me to sleep!" I beg them.

Someone places a mask over my mouth and tells me to breathe. They miss my mouth and the mask is half covering my eye and cheek. I struggle, attempting to show them,

"I can't breathe! Please! Help!"

The person holding the mask is busy, franticly yelling at the person across the room, and does not heed me. Instead, I am pressed harder into the table, and my scalp is smashed into the cold, hard table beneath it.

"Please! Just please!" I yell.

Immediately, a kind-faced nurse comes into view and adjusts my mask. "You are going to have to calm down."

"The pain! My God! Help me!"

She says nothing in return. Two people beside me are arguing that certain tests were not performed, and they will not put me to sleep. I begin to scream in pain, begging for my life. I scream until I am hoarse, until the back of my head begins to throb from being thrown onto the table, until I am put to sleep.

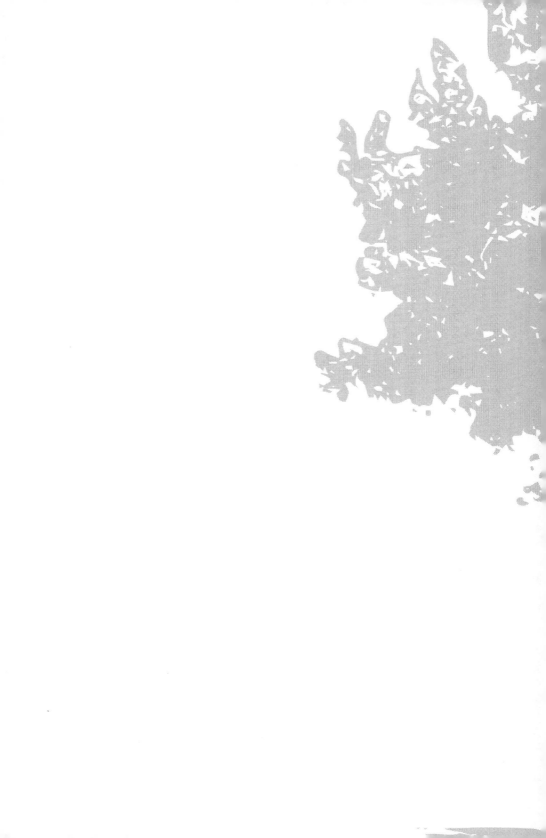

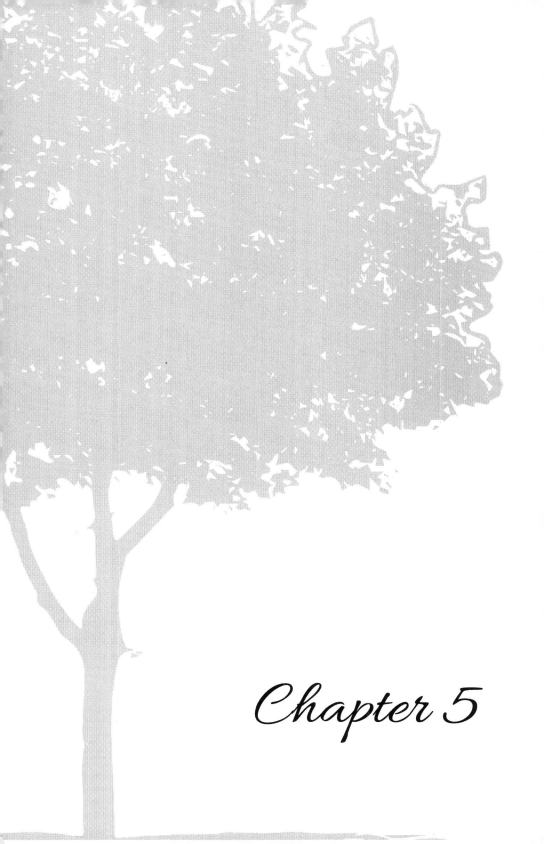

Chapter 5

Alive!

My first sensation upon waking up was hearing Matthew and the female nurse chatting.

"You should start to see her open her eyes from time to time," the nurse said.

"Okay," came Matthew's voice next.

I drifted back into unconsciousness. It was easier to stay asleep. I was ripped back into life by the sensation of a tube running down my throat. Suddenly, I cannot breathe, the hard, plastic tube screaming sensation running down my throat and deep inside my body. It hurt all way into my chest. I could feel wires and tubes running inside my body. I felt held down like my limbs were filled with lead. Terror consumed me. This tube running down my throat is consuming and panicking me. I gagged and sputtered. I could feel hot tears run down my cheeks, but could not wake up.

"NURSE!" It was Matthew again. "Nurse! For God's sake! She is choking!"

Back drifting in the medical dream world between awake and asleep. The sensations ease.

Hot tears, I feel them burning down my face. That damned tube in my throat wakes me and I hear Matthew once more.

"Okay, gumdrop. Look, you have to focus on breathing. Just breathe. In. Out. In. Out. They are going to take that damned tube out but you have keep breathing or they will put it back in. I am here." His finger is stroking the bridge of my nose like a cat. His skin is warm. I want to wrap my arms around his neck and smell him, but I am trapped. The tubes are all I can feel, and this weird, foggy sleep lures me back in again as I drift away from him into the murky fog of sleep.

Time passes.

"Melissa!" It is Matt. His voice is urgent and harsh.

I gasp. There is no tube in my throat. I feel the air rush into my mouth. All I can taste is its remnants, but no tube.

"Gumdrop, breathe! Try, just try to breathe." I hear the room full of nurses and doctors. I know I am alive. I know this is my new reality as I drift away once more.

I slowly open my eyes and see Matthew is at the foot of my bed. His head is down and he is glancing at his smartphone. In the corner, the TV is blaring about the government breakdown in Egypt. There are riots on the TV and a quiet in the room. I glance back at my darling Matthew and see he is not alone. Beside him is my brother.

"Oh. Shit. This is bad," is my first conscious thought. Chris left. He went back home after the baby shower and now he is back. His broad shoulders sit strong beside Matthew. Matt is not alone. It is okay. Chris' arms are crossed and his eyes are closed, his head resting back against the wall behind him. He looks like Dad, sitting like that. It amuses me just how much that would bug him.

I allow myself to drift in and out of consciousness. I hear the nurses bring Matthew coffee, and I am aware that my parents are coming soon. My brother is smack talking at the foot of my bed, always bravado, always attitude; Chris loves to poke fun and get a rise out of people.

I look down the end of my bed and see his lips moving and know he is just being ... Chris.

"Jackass," I say meekly from my position in the bed.

Matthew and Chris look up and see my eyes wide and awake.

"She's alive!" Chris mocks. "Yes! She is alive!" he laughs and I see the twinkle in his eyes.

Matthew and I do not need to say much. He comes to my side, takes my hand and instantly, we are united.

"Hi, blue eyes," I whisper, my voice horse and weak.

"Hey, you."

"What day is it?"

"It is Friday, babe." Matt looks drawn.

"I have been gone ..."

"... For three days."

Our silence speaks the volumes our hearts cannot. Three days. He pulls his chair up to me and sits beside me. He has dark circles around his eyes and is wearing the same clothes he was when we were separated. His hands are rough from the cold as they get in the winter months. Has he been wearing his gloves? His hands get windburn easily. I find myself consumed with thoughts of wanting to help him.

I never ask him the sex of the baby. I know wholeheartedly: a girl. I have just spent the last three days with her in a dream world of sorts, where I held her and begged for her forgiveness. Where I explained I had to return to her Daddy, and that I loved her so very much, as does her Daddy. In this dream world, I remember the warm, yellow light surrounding her and I, as I loved her, kissed her, and begged her goodbye for three days. Where I memorized her face, breathed in her skin, and kissed her a thousand times.

I want to tell Matthew about my three days with our girl, but I hardly have the words. I want to tell him that she is safe and loved, that I put her in the arms of my deceased Uncle, and heard him promise to love her, and then I kissed her goodbye. Matthew tells me that he got to see her, and I do not ask any more details. Right now, it is hard to even lift my fingers to hold his hand. I am profoundly weak and aware of my condition. Looking around, there are many poles at the head of my bed. My arms are covered in IV's.

There are four I can see from my position in bed, and I can feel the central line in my neck pulling if I move. My abdomen is draped and covered and I can tell by how the nurses move and support me that I am a mess under there.

I don't think I even want to know.

There are leg compressors on my legs that periodically go off to keep the blood moving. They hurt like blood pressure cuffs and wake me from my sporadic sleep. I am weak and ruined. That is enough for now. I know she is waiting to "meet" me, here on earth. I know I will have to face the fact my daughter is dead. But right now, in this bed, this is enough for me to understand.

Where are my parents? It feels like it has been hours of the three of us. Chris has left to eat and returned. Matt will not leave my side unless told to go, and Chris has already tried once. Just when I am about to ask, I hear them in the hall. Seeing their faces is a welcomed relief. I immediately see how worn they are. Oh, heavy hearts. Mom comes up and kisses my face. She is anxious and stays near. Her hands shake and I feel fear all over her. Dad embraces me, and then takes a chair and sits at the foot of the bed. He hangs onto my right foot and turns the television to the soccer channel. There is a familiarity in his touch. I am instantly comforted. The 8-year-old inside me wants to rip out the tubes and curl up on his chest and in his arms and have him tell me it will all be okay.

I know it won't, though. She is dead. I am in ruins, and so is my family. Lying in that bed, it becomes so clear exactly how ruined we all are. Yet, I cannot lift my arms. I cannot help. I am a victim of this horrid disorder, whatever this HELLP is. So I quietly close my eyes and hope they have the strength to carry me a while more.

That first day in the ICU, I drift in and out of sleep. The medications have a strong pull and I find myself riding a wave of chemicals and exhaustion. Doctors rotate in and out of my room. I see familiar faces, and the motorbike-jacket-wearing doctor returns without his bike gear. He smiles quietly and does not say a word as he quietly checks my chart and leaves. There are many faces I do not know, yet my family does. Social workers, doctors, and nurses all have an ease that I am completely new to, although, they know every intimate detail of my condition and care. It is jarring and unsettling.

My pain is increasing. With each leg compression and movement, the nurses make me down hot pain rips across my abdomen. I ask for help with the pain. A white-haired doctor with a stern face comes in and prescribes me narcotics, after asking a series of questions. He lets me know that I will be closely monitored and about the addictions risk involved. Having worked in Social Services, I know the facts and simply ask for the pain to be helped. He prescribes me opiates and leaves.

It is supper time and my family leaves for the night. Matthew has been brought a cot, and he has bedded down beside me for the night. We rest quietly, while the night nurse, Yolanda, drifts in and out. She has soft tears in her eyes, and she treats me gently and with great compassion. I am grateful for her.

In the morning, Matthew is somber. I can see the look in his eye that tells me he is preparing himself, and I know what for. My brother has arrived for the day and says that he has to go home today. I tell him I understand. He has been away from his family all week. He has a job and life to return to. Part of me is sad to see him go, yet I am beginning to tire of having everyone sitting and staring at me all the time. When he leaves, it will be one less set of eyes.

My parents arrive for the day and appear shaken. They stand united by the door to my room, and I know what is coming next; it is time.

Mom takes a deep breath and looks at me, and says, "Melissa, you need to meet her."

My mind races. It has been four days since her birth. I cannot bear to see her if her body is breaking down. I cannot have her be ruined. She is perfection. The girl I spent three days with in my mind is perfection.

"Will it ... is she ... gruesome?" I ask, my voice cracking and eyes welling with tears. I cannot handle the idea of her physical death on top of all the other deaths I am suffering.

"No. She is perfect," Mom says firmly. "Your Dad and I saw her this morning." Dad is quiet, behind her, and I see his pain.

"Okay."

Matthew pulls his chair next to the bed and we say nothing as my parents go to the morgue to get our daughter for us. Matt helps me put the head of the bed up so I can see better, though I am so weak, I know I cannot hold her. I can barely lift my arms. How will I not drop her?

My parents come into the room and Matthew goes to them. She is dressed in a dark pink sleeper and light hat. Matt tenderly takes her in his arms and sits down on the bed beside me. I feel my parents sink into the corner of the room, trying to give us space and quiet together as a family of three.

"Here she is," Matt says quietly.

I glance over at her and I know her face. In a flash, my three days with her floods back, where she was alive and bright and beautiful and vibrant. In the coma, she was whole, where I held her sweet warm body and breathed in her scent. With Matthew snuggled in next to me so I could best see her, I reached across to pull down the blanket that she was wrapped in. As I did so, I felt the radiating cold coming off her body.

Every cell in my body screamed. I felt terror run through me. Cold. She is ice cold. She is dead and cold and not what I remember. I felt the bile rise in my throat and my nerves beginning to undo. I wanted to scream and rip every damned tube out of my body in the horror of it. I want to scream. I want to rip this room to shreds. Why? Why is her body different than I remember?

Death.

Taking a deep breath, and then another, I closed my eyes for a moment. This is my only moment on this earth with her. I know it is. I need to do this. I steady myself and dig deep within me.

Regaining composure, I focused my eyes on her little hat. What a sweet little hat! I stared at her face, careful not to touch her skin too much. If I felt that cold again, I may not be able to be present. I may very well drift into insanity.

She has my nose. My inward sweeping button nose. And my hands. Matthew's eyes. She is simply gorgeous. Looking at Matthew holding her, it becomes apparent; he has become a father while I slept. He holds her close. The cold doesn't seem to be bothering him.

I keep willing her eyes to open. I will her to breathe. She is completely still. Not like the baby I held.

The room is silent. All eyes are on me. I stare at my wee girl and sigh. I know it is time to let her go. In my medicated haze, I drink in the sight of her face and say goodbye for what will be the second of a hundred times.

Putting my head back on my pillow, I tell Matthew I am okay. My parents come and take her from Matthew's arms, and leave quietly with her. There is nothing to say.

The chaos of the hospital sweeps into our room slowly. It is obvious that the nurses were holding off their rotations to allow us to have some quiet time with our girl. However, they cannot be held back for long. Soon, it is time for in-bed x-rays, blood work, and more observers standing at the foot of my bed. They come in on the hour for something new: to change my sheets or change my pads. Fluid is pouring out of me now. I sweat through sheets in hours, and my entire intestinal system is in revolt. The stream of people and physical touching is endless. Matthew is called in and out of the room, depending on procedures, and we are both growing weary of the hospital game. It is apparent we have much more to go.

I am very weak. I cannot even lift my arms to move the hair from my eyes. Matthew is given a welcome reprieve to leave the hospital a while and goes home to my parents' to sleep. He is simply exhausted, my long night of hallucinations keeping him up with me, and although he does not want to leave, he does so under my parents' advisement.

While he is gone, I ask my Mom if Kath is coming. She says she is and that she will come later that day.

Mom says she has brought some supplies for me to feel better. Face wash, makeup, hair pins, and lotion. She begins to unpack the bag to take care of me. Her hands feel welcomed after the clinical hands of the day all poking and prodding me. She has to move carefully around me, as she navigates the poles of tubes that are attached to me. She rubs lotion in my skin and I begin to feel anew.

She says she is going to do my hair next. My big, thick, shoulder-length, curly hair, which has taken on a life of its own in the hospital bed. She takes out a bristled brush and begins to brush. My hair reacts to this in one way and one alone: sheer frizz. I cringe, knowing that this will only make the situation worse, and not better.

But she is trying so hard to help me feel better. Her hands are shaking from the anxiety that has rained down on us for over a week. I let her brush and brush until I am sure my hair stands a foot wide on each side.

Just then, my sister walks in the room. We have that sisterly communication with our eyes,

"Dear Lord, what is she doing with your hair?"

"Help! But be nice."

Mom is braiding it back off of my face and Kath takes my hand at the side of the bed.

"Hey, squirt," she says: one of my many childhood nicknames.

We small chat and Mom takes leave from the room after finishing the braid.

"Help this!" I say to Kath as we giggle, her rebraiding and adjusting the mess on top of my head.

"I think it unsalvageable. We may have to shave you bald, kid." She pulls and tugs and I am instantly reminded of the hours of torture being her hairstylist victim.

"Shut up and just fix it."

As she pulls and tugs, I sit quiet. How am I here now? Isn't my sister supposed to be showing me how to change her diaper? The shock of what has happened to us courses through my body, and I am suddenly overwhelmed with it all.

Kath is done fixing my hair, and I hear her talking as she sifts through her bag. She, too, has brought comfort items to help me feel better. She says that she is going to get me something nicer to wear than the hospital gowns, and I am grateful. A lull happens in the conversation and she approaches the bed and takes my hand. Our eyes lock. Fatigue washes over me—these damned meds—the shock and chaos are overtaking me once more.

"I am sorry, I am a bit of a one-trick pony right now, sis," I say weakly.

Her eyes twinkle and she laughs. "Yes, you are," she says with a smile.

Later that afternoon, Matthew returns and we prepare for another long night in the Intensive Care Unit. After begging all day for food, they brought me a clear fluid diet to eat. Within one spoon of the broth, I am instantly nauseated. It tastes like broth from a powder, and after five days completely empty, my stomach revolts. I push it away and sip on the off-brand ginger ale. It does not taste quite right either, but at least settles in my belly better.

Matthew has a cot sitting in the side of the room, and some of the nurses have brought him reading material. I see him staring through the pages without seeing. It occurs to me that it has been hours since he has arrived. Past supper time. He must be hungry as well.

"Babe, you should eat," I say meekly.

"I am not leaving you," his tone flat, nonnegotiable.

"I will be fine. Just run and get a sandwich and come back."

"The family has all gone home for the day. I am not leaving."

I drop it for another half an hour. I know better than to push him when his mind is set so.

Our new nurse comes in and says she will be with us for the night. An older lady, no-nonsense. She reminds me of a stern, semi-retired supply teacher. I instantly miss my day-shift nurses. As night is for sleeping, so surely I will not have to deal with her much.

She says she will get me my meds, and hopefully, I can get some sleep. She leaves the room to get my medication.

I turn my face to Matthew,

"Matt, babe..." I look at him in all earnest.

"Okay. Fine. 10 minutes. I will be right back. I have my cell phone." He kisses the bridge of my nose and leaves.

Settling into the quiet, I hear my door open. Looking up, I see a small-statured, beautiful nurse. Her long hair is piled on the top of her head, and I can see the tears in her eyes. She is not the first nurse to cry, and I find myself comforted in their tears.

"Hi, I am Nancy. I am a nurse here. I am working elsewhere, but I just had to come in and say hello." I can hear the pain in her voice as she approaches the bed. "I just ... I don't know what to say." She wrings her hands. "I have two kids and I just cannot imagine. I just cannot imagine losing ..." Her voice breaks off.

"Thank you," I reply. I am confused. What am I supposed to say? Thank you feels wrong. Thank you for talking about my dead child? Thank you for your children being alive and mine not? I realize she is talking and I cannot hear her. Lost in my own thoughts, I shake my head and attempt to listen,

"... you are doing really well. You are so strong. I cannot imagine what you are going through."

"Thank you," I find myself saying again. What do I say? I do not understand. Why do some children live and mine did not? This new existence makes no sense! An angry fire burns in my belly and sadness bites the back of my throat. I just do not understand.

"It is okay," I find myself saying. Wait, what? Why am I comforting her? Seeing her upset, I want to comfort her. This is backwards! "It is okay, really."

"I will let you rest. I will come back and check on you later if I can."

I am touched that she came out of her way, which she knew of what happened to us and wanted to give condolences. But I have no idea how to receive them. I find myself confused and saddened. What do you say to others' pity of your life? Am I pitied now?

Without warning, the stern nurse comes back in and hands me my medication. Her eyes are fixed on me as I take the narcotics. I feel small and common, suddenly.

"I am sorry; I know you told me, what is your name again?" I ask.

"Constance."

"Thank you, Constance" I say, returning my medication cup, empty.

She leaves me in peace for ten minutes, to get sleep, as they always say. Sleep is futile. The hallway is filled with activity and noise. She returns to empty my catheter bag. She sits the jug on the floor and picks up the bag to empty it into the jug. As she does so, my catheter pulls hard.

"Ouch!" I exclaim. My hands fly to my groin. "Please stop! That hurts."

She looks up at me from the floor with a look of irritation. "Alright."

"Oh," she says, "Your catheter is coming out. I need to reseat it."

Fear floods me. The last catheter I had was the cervical catheter at the Catholic hospital. The one that left me screaming in agony as my cervix was ripped open in an attempt to get labor moving.

And this urinary catheter would be no different. Searing, hot, pain ripped through me. Powerless and too weak to fight her off, I begged her to stop. She said she had to reinsert it and if I would just lie still, it would all be over. The room was dark. I looked at the door, begging for Matthew to come back.

The pain narcotic begins to kick in. I could feel the fog rising slowly from the floor, encapsulating the bed. Please, make the pain stop. She fiddled and pulled, yanked and ripped at me. I saw her gloved hands with blood on them as she said she was done. Throbbing, pulsating pain, I pulled my blankets over my groin, and held myself and cried.

Matthew returned to see me curled up in a ball, sobbing, in agony from the mutilating "reseating" of my catheter.

"I was only gone 10 fucking minutes!" His exasperation filled the room as he got onto the bed and wrapped his strong arms around me. I weep like a child into the crook of his arm, shaking so hard, I can hear the bed rattle, and I feel his hot tears on my neck. "Who did this to you? Tell me now!"

I tell him her name. He leaves. I never see her again.

Night two, consciousness in the Intensive Care Unit is harrowing and terrifying. Next door, an emergency case is brought in and there is a flurry of activity. Noise, loud shouting family members, and a patient who screams of anguish keep Matthew and I awake all night. Sleep deprivation, a nightmare reality, all mix with narcotics, and I hallucinate spiders crawling the walls of my room, screaming patients, agony, and terror. I spend a fitful night lost in terror and hallucination. At night, all the monsters come out and I am in anguish.

By morning, Matthew and I are purely exhausted. I have kept him up all night in my terror, confusion, and constant requests for comfort. By the time the sun rises, we look as if we were worse than ever before. Once the sun rises, the monsters ease and we rest, as much as possible with the constant comings and goings of hospital staff, nurses, and doctors. When we finally wake, some time past breakfast, the warm February sun is streaming into my room. I look out and see the bright sun for the first time in days and am completely relieved. Life is present.

I roll over in bed and see that Matt looks simply exhausted. I am infuriated with this existence. I want out of this ICU. Shifting in my bed, I feel the wires pull. Fed up, I raise the head of my bed and begin to look around the room. A clarity washes over me, my anger empowering me. Where am I? What am I dealing with, exactly? I look around the room and see that I have two poles attached to my bed. One is attached to this line that is running to my neck, the other is running to my IV in my arm. Okay. Two poles down from four; that is something. I look behind me and see the blood pressure cuff reader. I have had a blood pressure cuff on constantly since I woke. Okay, two poles and a blood pressure cuff. I uncover my legs and see that they are no longer wrapped in pressure bandages. I look at my toes. They look skinny. Why do my toes look skinny? Have I lost weight? I yank up my dressing gown and see that, in fact, my legs are thinner, and there are now faint purple stretch marks on the back of my knees. Weird. I must have gained weight rapidly and lost it.

Why?

I shake my head. Come on, think, Melissa! I feel like I am trying to shake out the cobwebs. Why would you have gained weight in a coma? Water? Swelling! I must have swelled in the coma. Okay. And now I have lost the swelling and apparently the weight with it. I run my hands over my arms and wrists and feel the bones are more prominent. I look down at my belly and it is swollen like a balloon; I still look 8 months pregnant. I touch my stomach cautiously and feel a thick wrap around the incision under my breasts. It is like a tensor bandage. My stomach feels loose, almost jelly-like underneath it. My stomach is empty. I have no baby, I remind myself. She is dead.

Covering myself back up, I observe the rest of the room. I am in a glass-walled room. It is smaller than I thought. There are curtains that cover the glass walls. That is why it appears sunny sometimes and not at others.

Outside in the corridor, I can see my nurse at her station. She is pretending not to be watching me as I look around. My IV and line in my neck hurt, pull, and tug. I am uncomfortable and fidgeting as she walks into the room.

"Good morning," I say. It is Zee, the same day nurse that I had yesterday. I like her. She is concise and professional, but still warm. I point to Matt sleeping and put my finger to my lips. She approaches the bed and puts her ear to my lips.

"I want out of here," I say ardently. "How do I get out of the ICU?"

She smiles and laughs at my forwardness. "Well, that is a start. Why don't we try and get you up and about today? Maybe sit in the chair a little later?"

"Yes! Can I try to eat again? I am hungry."

"Of course. The doctors are going to do their rounds shortly. Why don't you try and rest? I hear you had a rough night. Once they are done rounds, we will bring you something to eat." She leaves the room quietly and pulls the curtain behind her.

Rest. I do not want to rest. I want out of this place. I lower the head of my bed and try to curl up, but the wires and IV lines pull and make getting comfortable nearly impossible. I pull the blankets up to my face and try and close my eyes awhile.

Sleep is good and peaceful. I am awoken by the feeling of someone in my room. I open my eyes to see the dark-haired, handsome, motor-bike-driving doctor at the foot on my bed.

"Hello," I say.

"Hello," he responds in a thick, Spanish accent.

"I know you..."

"Yes, you do," he smirks. "Rest now."

There is something calming and comforting about his presence. I wish he could stay. I close my eyes and hear him leave.

A while later, I wake again to find a short-statured, older man standing at the foot of my bed. He is a doctor, dressed in scrubs and white coat. I smile at him and the warmth in his smile back fills the room. I hear Matt chatting quietly with him. He comes over and places his hand on Matt's shoulder and they joke. He leaves and I turn to Matt.

"Who was that?"

"The head of Obstetrics."

"Ha! I bet we have his attention"

"No kidding. Nice guy. He has come every day to see you."

"He has? Where was he before?"

"Not there. But he is here now."

I pull the blankets up and wonder, what if he had been there? Was he supposed to be there? I laid in bed, writhing for mercy from a doctor for hours and no relief was found until shift change, so maybe if he was there ... the miles of what ifs unravel in my mind. I am interrupted by Zee returning to the room with a breakfast tray.

"I found you some food! Care to get out of bed and have a bite?"

"Out of bed?" Matt's voice drips with shock and concern.

"Yes," I beam with excitement. "Get me out of this damned bed." I look at him and see a little fear behind his eyes. I nod, attempting to reassure him that I want this.

Zee takes time setting up the room. She moves the chair from the corner of the room next to the bed. I know what she is doing because I have done the same in my care for the disabled, and I was taught these same lifts and techniques. Humbling to now be having them done on me.

She moves the table and my breakfast tray far out of the way and comes over.

"I am going to put my arms under your arms. You are going to stand up on your feet. Once you are ready, shuffle one foot at a time and I will turn you into your chair. Don't worry about the wires. I will take care of them. Okay?"

"Yup." I take a deep breath. I know what she needs me to do, as I have done this before when caring for clients. I can do this.

I feel her lift me up under my arms and I am on my feet. Immediately, my knees buckle under my own weight. Oh, Lord! I am so weak. I lean into her, as I have felt clients do hundreds of times before. This is humiliating! I feel anger burn down my throat. Screw this! I summon every ounce of strength and push down and firmly stand on my knees. Ha! I am standing.

"Good job, Melissa!" Zee breathes into my neck. "Okay, one step at a time."

We slowly shuffle over to the chair and she eases me into my chair. I look up at her and she smiles warmly at me. "You did it!"

And it felt good.

She brings over my tray and tells me to take my time eating. I glance down at my tray and see the usual suspects. Jell-O, juice, some crackers, and ginger ale. I am still on a fluids-only diet. Sigh. Baby steps.

Matt comes over. "Well, look at you!" His smile is broad. He is proud of me and I beam back at him. "Progress, right, gumdrop? Take it easy, okay?"

"Are you hungry?" I ask

"Yeah. I may go get a bite somewhere. Are you okay?"

I assure him that I am just fine with my Jell-O and ask him to bring me the remote for the television to keep me company. He leaves and I find myself renewed. I nibble slowly at my Jell-O. My tummy is hungry, and I can hear it rumbling. I actually want to eat, but I am taking it slow. I am scared of vomiting with these incisions. That seems nightmarish. Ghoulish, in fact.

I barely have a chance to contemplate my circumstances before the next round of activity waves into the room. Blood work this time, then an ultrasound technician will be coming later.

"Oh yay, me," I mutter as they leave me to my half-eaten Jell-O and juice. The tests just keep coming. I need to find out why they are testing me, what are these tests for? As I begin to come out of the fog, I realize how little I know about my own condition. Maybe this is why they always ask for next of kin?

Matt returns with my parents in tow. They are joking about slipping in the back entrance of the unit. I forget that, although, it feels like I just got here, I have been here six days now.

"Hey! Look at you." Mom's smile is warm and across her face, seeing me sitting in a chair.

"Not bad, right?" I conjure a smile back. My face doesn't feel like it is mine.

Dad comes over and glances down at my food tray. "You need to eat."

"I know, Dad." I glance up at him. Dad, his kids, and their food. It makes my Dad's skin crawl to think his kids do not have enough to eat or are hungry. Not as in a stereotypical way, but rather, genuine distress if he thinks his kids are not eating enough. My stomach feels raw and I cannot fathom taking another bite. I try and redirect his attention.

"Hey, Dad, is there any soccer on?"

His glance tells me that my tactics were noted. "No, it is Sunday." I see the smirk under his mustache.

The next round of testing comes through, with a shift change later that afternoon. I spend the day napping, chatting and listening to my family joke about my urine bag ("Oh! That is good pee! Look at that pee!"), poking good natured fun at me from the end of the bed.

Mid-afternoon, my midwife Laura comes in. I hear her voice before I see her enter the room. My heart swells and I feel like every cell in my body could explode. Laura! She came. I reach earnestly out of my bed for her hand and we lock grip and eyes.

"Hey, you." Her voice gentle and rasped.

"Oh, Laura."

"Look at you. Huh? Gave us quite the scare." Her eyes burrowing into mine. She is worried. I feel her grip on me tighten and I feel her ache.

"I didn't know if you would come."

"Of course I would come..."

"Though I imagine you were exhausted." I remember that she crusaded for us all night long.

Bits and pieces of our time together from that day begin to flow back to me on the sound of her voice. The chaos of the room, the doctor's face, Matt's fear, my baby. *My baby.*

"Did you see her? Melissa, she is beautiful." I am slammed back to reality. "Yes. Yes I did. I was able to spend some time yesterday. Mom and Dad brought her to me."

Laura stands by my bedside for some time, observing the family, not once letting go of my hand. I feel as if she could crawl in bed with me for hours and stay there. I want her to. My beautiful Laura. I wish I could just keep her by my side.

"It is okay, Melissa, to grieve." Those green eyes are on me again. She proceeds to tell me of the power of hope and a beautiful story that she read of the belief that a baby will come again, come to this earth until it gets to stay. It is the first time since waking that I am given permission to grieve her and I feel myself thawing, as if from a great frozen time. I do not feel safe to grief here. I need to fight to live. I soak in her words like roots in the rain and pray that I have the strength for them later.

I am growing weary. Laura notices my fatigue and takes her leave after promising to return. After closing my eyes a while, I hear the family drift out to let me rest. A little later, I hear my afternoon nurse, Sandy, in my room once more, and I open my eyes to find her looking at me.

"I was wondering," I ask softly, "how much longer I have to be here. When will I be out of the ICU?"

"Funny you should say that," she smiles, "we were supposed to move you up this afternoon, but we are just waiting for a room."

I glance at Matt. His eyes brighten. No more ICU. Okay! Let's do this.

"One of the things we have to do, however, is to remove your central line." She points to the line that is in my neck. "So let me get my things together and we will get that taken out."

I look at Matt and feel nervous. What is this now? I bring my hand up to my neck and feel the large tube line that is feeding into my neck. I imagine this is going to be interesting.

She comes in and begins to prep her area. Matt and I are chatting. He is trying to distract me by putting grossly inappropriate stand-up comedy on the television. It works. We laugh and glance at each other, and wonder what those around us must be thinking as we listen to this smut in the ICU. And yet, neither of us care.

She comes over and begins to work on the line. She then asks Matt to come over to the bed. Matt takes my hand.

"This is going to feel a little weird. When I say, take a deep breath, okay?"

Oh God. This is going to suck. When nurses say something is weird, it is always so much worse than weird.

"I have to take a deep breath? What's to breathe for?" I mutter to Matt as she works.

"Okay, deep breath in."

I summon my courage and take the deepest breath I can muster. This bizarre, ripping, crawling sensation goes through my upper chest. Up to my clavical and through my neck, I feel this long tube come out of my body. It is, by far, one of the weirdest and most awful bodily sensations I have ever had. I gasp for breath, half-panicked, as Matt grips my hand.

"I gotcha. I gotcha," he says calmly.

"What the...!"

"That was a particularly long one," Nurse Sandy says. She holds it up for Matt to see, and I can see by his expression that I do not want to turn around and see what came out of me. She quietly stitches me up and chuckles at the comedy that is still on the TV.

"Not long now, and we should be able to move you upstairs," she says with a smile as she leaves the room.

Matt is as relaxed as I think I have seen him. He is curled up on his cot, his magazines stacked at the end of it, and chuckling at the TV. I lower my bed closer to the ground and reach out my arm to him. We hold hands. Slowly regrouping, I feel my body relax.

Sandy returns and says it is time to go. She seems to be rushing, suddenly. Perhaps they need my room for someone else. What a sad thought that is. I could not be more eager to transfer out of my ICU bed and onto the bed that would take me upstairs. Matt grabs our stuff and I see him carefully place a white square box under his arm. What is in that white box? I do not remember seeing that before. We make our way down the halls, and the nurses joke together. Leaving the loud, constant brightness of the ICU, behind the halls outside of it are quiet. I hear stillness for the first time in a very long time. They wheel me onto an elevator and press for floor 7.

"The Neurology floor?" Matt questions.

He knows this hospital well. I am surprised. The Neurology floor is for stroke and dementia patients. I look up at him, confused. I guess it is better than being on a maternity floor.

"It was the only spot that had a private room. We wanted you guys to have your own space," the nurse explained.

Matt and I share a look. Okay. Neurology it is. I feel like I am on the edge of sanity anyways, so it seems ironically fitting.

The elevator bings and the doors open. It is the evening, and the floor is dark and quiet. As they wheel me quickly down the halls, I crane my neck to see just where I am going. Door after door shows ward rooms with two or three beds in each. All quiet with the patients asleep. We stop at the nurses' station, and they direct us to the end of the hall. Friendly-faced and warm, I instantly relax at the sight of them. I feel safe.

They wheel my bed into the final room at the end of a long corridor. It is so quiet, I feel like I should whisper, and the quiet rings. They help me transfer out of the bed and into the ward bed in the room. It is thin and hard. My ICU bed was much more comfortable, but this bed hurts the moment I touch it. The room is cold, almost like it was shut and waiting for us. One of my new nurses, Janet, brings me a warm blanket and water.

"Have you had anything to eat, my love?" She smiles warmly.

"They had me on a fluid-only diet. I am hungry."

"Oh, they do not have food down there. Let me bring you a few nibbles to get you through the night."

She brings me ginger ale, crackers, and a cookie. She hands a cookie to Matt with a wink. "Now just press this button here," she said, pointing to the call button, "If you need me." She leaves the room and a silence falls.

Matt looks at me and chuckles.

"It is crazy quiet here."

"I know!" Our thoughts aligned completely.

Matt folds out his cot and gets himself settled. I see him gently place the white box up on the shelf above his cot.

I look around and attempt to get my bearings. A small room with a corridor cupboard. I saw the bathroom in the hallway on the way in. My bed is facing a wall with a large curtain. Matt sees me staring at them and goes over to open them. We have a wall-to-wall window facing out from the 7th floor, looking out at the city and the local University.

"Oh, wow. Room with a view, ma'am." I see a twinkle in his eye.

"They must have wanted us to have a nice space to recover in," I bemuse.

"Agreed. That was kind of them."

Matt settles onto his cot, and I nibble on my snacks. Food feels good. The quiet feels incredible and slightly unsettling. Nurse Janet returns with my medication. She hands me the narcotics with an earnest smile. I stare at them a moment and relent. I hate these stupid drugs. I really do not want another night of terror. But they keep giving them to me, so I must need them. I have to do what they say.

After she is gone, Matt and I settle in for the night. I ask him to leave the curtains open so I can see the city lights. It is grounding in the chaos.

The lights are off, and I hear Matt drift away, sleeping. I feel lightheaded and feel the bed floating. Afraid to close my eyes, I try and focus on the window as long as I can. Suddenly, I am asleep and I hear screams rip down the hall.

I gasp awake. Was that my scream? Who is in terror? Oh, good heavens, what was that?

I shake and pull the blankets under my chin. Spiders crawl across the ceiling, screaming rips through my mind, and I look down to see blood seeping out from underneath my bed.

Horror! Again. Not again, this will not happen again. I have had enough. I reach out, trembling to turn on the bedside light. I need something. I need help. *I need help.* I need someone who can help me. I need someone I can trust to fix this. I need someone who knows what to do. I can't stand just one more second of this. I am so terrified, I quake until my teeth rattle and I shiver uncontrollably. *Help me.* Who can I trust?

I need my midwives.

I look over at Matt sleeping and I cannot reach the phone. His cellphone is on the bedside table, but I cannot reach it because my catheter is tied to the end of the bed. I reach out my hand and try, but my catheter yanks and I screech out in pain. Matt stirs,

"Matt, babe."

"Hm..."

"Matt, babe. I am sorry. I need the phone."

"The phone? What?" He sits up, confused and half-awake. "Why do YOU need the phone?"

"Because I need the phone," I said, my eyes staring firmly back at his. "I need this to end and I need to talk to someone who will know what to do."

"Okay." I can tell he is still confused, but he hands me back the phone and lays back down.

I search through his contacts and find the midwives' number and dial.

In the middle of the night, they have a call-answering service. I tell the person my name, which team of midwives care for me, and telephone number. I hang up the phone and wait for the return call. Sitting with the side light on, I cannot see the hallucinations quite so clearly. Something about the dark makes them worse. Matt puts a t-shirt over his eyes and rests. After a few long minutes, the phone rings.

"Hello."

"Hello, Melissa? It is Jill."

I breathe a sigh of relief. I adore Jill. She helped me when I felt like my water broke. She is logical, down to earth, and has common sense. She is exactly who I need in this moment.

"Jill. Thank goodness it is you. I know this is going to sound crazy but I need you to help me think straight."

"What is going on?"

"They have me on this medication. For pain. It makes me hallucinate at night. It is horrible. The walls..." My voice cracking with fear. "They crawl with bugs. It is awful. I do not know what do it."

"Are you in any pain?"

"No."

"On a one to ten scale, any pain at all?"

"I hurt. I am sore, but not bad. Not like the shoulder pain. This is manageable."

"Okay." I hear her take a deep breath. "You can ask to go off of the medication. You have that right."

"I do?"

"Yes. Yes, you do. You can refuse the medication. If you think the hallucinations are being caused by them, tell your nurse you do not want that medication anymore, and they will have to stop it."

Listening to her words, I find myself sitting straight up in bed. I am hanging on her every word. I can just ask them to stop the medication? I can just ask them to stop the medication! I feel myself stand up inside of myself. I can just do this. I can just take charge and do this. This ends now.

"Thank you, Jill. Thank you. I just didn't know. I feel so confused. I can't think straight and I know I am not coping with no sleep ..." Tears pour hotly down my cheeks.

"I know, honey. You have been through a hell of an ordeal. I could hardly believe it was your number calling. I thought, with all the nurses, why would you need me?"

"I just needed someone I could trust. I needed someone who I knew could help me."

"Anytime. Anytime. Do you want me to talk to the nurses for you?"

"Could you, please?"

"I will let them know your request and they will follow up with you, okay?"

"Thank you, Jill."

I hang up the phone and feel a calm wash over me. Keeping the side light on, I lie back and watch out the window at the city lights. If I can refuse medication, I must have some control. Some control, when my life, my dignity, my existence has been dictated by the medical teams for so long. I have control? It doesn't feel like I have any say in anything. Confused, in a haze of medication, I am unable to reconcile these two things. My body is not my own anymore. I look down at my swollen belly and lift my gown. I see the bandage wrapping around my chest. It binds over my breasts. It makes me achy from being held still for so long. My thin legs stretch out before more. I am alive. I am ruined and alive. She is dead. I am alive. I shake my head. This just doesn't make sense.

Covering myself back up, anger builds in my belly. How did I get here? Hallucinating, lying in a hospital bed, nearly dead, and not nearly alive. This is such bullshit. I am done with this.

I roll over in bed and feel my catheter pull yet again. That, I decide, is the next thing to go. I want unchained from this bed. I am pissed. Enough already. Lying in the light of the side light, I decide to fight.

"Hey, baby girl, watch what Mama can do," I mutter into the darkness. "Mama's about to fight."

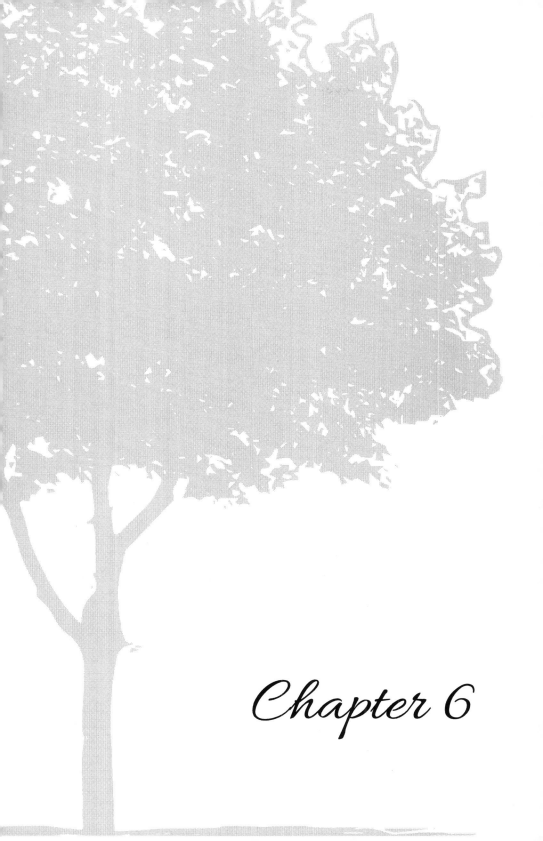

Chapter 6

Escape the Monster

I am awoken in the morning by the sound of the orderly coming into change the laundry bag.

Slam! Bang!

I look up from my bed, and see her back walking out of the room.

"Mornin' to you too," I grumble.

I hear Matt snicker. I look up to see his eyes on mine.

"Hi."

"Hey, you. How was last night?"

"Long, awful, and over. It changes today."

"What changes today?"

"This." I motion at my body in the bed. "All of this."

He nods. He is unsure what I mean, but his brain isn't quite turned on from sleep yet. That is okay. I do not need him awake yet.

Just then, an entire team of doctors come into the room. One resident leads the pack, with four minions following. They line up at the foot of my bed and stare at me. Startled, I sit up straight and try to fix my hair. Matt does the same and we stare at them like just-woken deer in headlights.

What time is it? I wonder. I glance at the clock: 7:15 am. Okay. I guess this is when the day gets started on floor 7.

The resident doctor begins to rattle off my medical conditions and pelt the minions with questions. They reply in kind. Matt and I glance uncomfortably at each other. Do we need to be here for this?

"How are you feeling, Melissa?"

Oh! That is me!

"Um. Okay. I guess."

"How is your pain? I see you have been prescribed narcotics."

"Yes. My pain is manageable. I no longer want the narcotics."

"Okay. Well, the narcotics are there to assist you..." I cut him off mid-sentence.

"I do not care. The pain is manageable. I do not want the narcotics." I can hear Jill's voice ring through my ears. "You have the right to refuse medication..."

The minions scribble in their notebooks. A gentle-faced, lanky, younger, male doctor at the back of the group is not writing. He stares at me kindly. I smile warmly at him. He is actually watching me. Bemused, I watch him back.

Just then, the Spanish-speaking, motorbike-jacket-wearing doctor from the ICU walks in. I recognize him; wait a minute, what is his name? My memory is so fuzzy.

I glance at Matthew and I see him relax. This doctor is good news. I sit back.

"Hello, Melissa. I am Dr. Hernandez. I operated on your liver. How are you feeling today?"

"I am good, I mean, I guess." There are now six sets of eyes staring at me from the end of my bed, and I cannot remember the last time I brushed my hair. Can I have a shower before we have this conversation? "I would like to be able to get up and move around. When can I get my catheter out?"

A bemused smile snakes across his face. I cannot tell what he is thinking, but I can tell I am not what he expected.

"I do not see why you cannot have your catheter out today. After rounds, we will have it removed."

"Melissa has denied any further narcotics." The resident perks up from behind Dr. Hernandez. His face turns expressionless.

"Why is this, Melissa?" he asks, his tone sweet and kind.

"Because I do not like them. They scare me. I hallucinate. I do not want them."

"We do not want you to be in pain..." His eyebrows raised. "You have had very significant surgery."

"I will tell you."

His bemused smirk returned. "Okay then. We can alternate acetaminophen and ibprophen to keep you comfortable. We need to send you for another CT scan ..."

He drifts off into doctor speak and I sense Matthew step forward. I did what I needed to. I am taking back control in baby steps. I am exhausted by of all this. I see Matthew talking it all over with the white coats at the end of the room and I check out. Matt has it.

"... I will come back at the end of the day to check on you and to discuss the results of the tests." I snap back into reality. He will be back, okay. That is a comfort. I find him reassuring and we have much more to discuss. Much more.

Dr. Hernandez leaves the room to continue his rounds, and we are left with the resident and his minions at the foot of my bed. The blank staring commences again.

"Oh," Matt says, "I was wondering, how is the fluid in her lungs?"

Fluid in my lungs? This is news.

"Fluid in her lungs?" The resident searches his chart, and the minions follow suit, as there is a mass shuffling of paper at the foot of my bed.

"Yes. They were doing daily x-rays in the ICU because there was a fluid build-up during the time of sedation." Matt is starting to sound like a doctor. "I was curious if it has all drained as they saw it going down, but we have yet to have confirmation."

"Well, we will need to x-ray her to make sure."

Great, another x-ray.

"We will need to get her down to x-ray right away, before adjusting her antibiotic amounts..." The doctors are scurrying at the end of my bed. They talk over each other, and one grabs for the phones while they shuffle through papers. Chaos suddenly envelops the room. I feel my brain begin to swim. No! No more chaos. I just want to have breakfast. I want to have breakfast, and wake up and be left alone.

One of the doctors comes over and starts to take my blood pressure. I do not remember him asking to touch me. I recoil and frown up at him. I hear Matt attempting to quiet the room, the anger in his voice is palpable. I reach out for Matt's hand, but he is at the foot of the bed, attempting to quiet the chaos.

"Please. Do not overwhelm her. Please! Can we not all come at her at once?" I hear his voice ardent.

Someone is taking my blood pressure while another asks a question of me. The room spins and I shut down.

I close my arms across my body and close my eyes.

Make it stop. Breathe. Make it stop. Breathe.

Matt's face is in mine. The room is empty, as he has gotten rid of the hoard. "Babe, we have to take you down for an x-ray. I am so sorry. It is all my fault. I shouldn't have said anything."

"What is happening to me?" Adrenaline is coursing through me. I taste metal and cannot slow down my heart. "No, it isn't your fault."

"They are sending an orderly. They will take you down. I will be right there."

I look down at my hands and realize that I am shaking like a leaf in the wind. Shaking so hard, I can hear the bed shake beneath me.

"Oh, I am so sorry." Matt wraps his big arms around me and I sob. "It is my fault. I shouldn't have told them. That resident. He wouldn't listen."

"Can you stay with me? The x-ray, where am I going? I am scared. What is this?"

"The other x-rays you had, you were in bed for them. They are refusing to let you have another one of those, and are sending you down to the second floor for it. They want you to go down to the department. But I worked in the department, right? I know everyone there. I will make this okay."

I shake in his arms. What just happened? I felt so good and now, I feel so bad. The walls feel like they are closing in on me and in just a matter of seconds.

An orderly comes in and tells me he is wheeling me down for an x-ray. It all happens so quickly. I just woke up a few moments ago! They wheel me down the same hallway that was so quiet last night. In the morning, it is busy and bustling. It is filled with people, giant breakfast carts, while confused patients wander the hall with their nurses. They stop my bed at the nurses' station by the elevator. I can hear a patient moaning in confusion. Her cries instantly nauseate and overwhelm me. I cannot think or breathe. All I can hear is her pain scream, her confusion much like mine. I cover my ears with my hands. I can barely stand it. The pain, it is everywhere, the chaos, my world has spun out of control.

The elevator dings and I am relieved to be taken away from that moment. On the x-ray floor, he lines me up with all the other patients in beds against a wall in the hallway. I am in full open view of the waiting room patients. I pull the blankets up over my breasts. I am only in a thin hospital gown. I am exposed and shaken to my core.

Matt's face is in mine once more. "Wait here, gumdrop. I will find out what is going on." He quickly leaves my side and I am terrified. I cling to my blankets and close my eyes like a child in a thunderstorm. Maybe if I just do not see it, I will not feel it.

Matt returns. His anger is less, though still palpable. He rubs my foot and tells me that Marg is going to help me. I remember his stories of Marg from his time working here. She is very good. Matthew has described her as knowledgeable, but not exactly the picture of warmth and compassion.

I look at his eyes and he reassures me that it will be okay.

Marg comes down the hall and tells Matt to bring me down. Matt pushes my hospital bed up to the x-ray room. The last x-ray room I remember being in was at the county hospital. Where she was still alive. Where I was in so much pain. This room is almost identical. Terror rips through me.

"Hello, Melissa." Marg's voice is soft. I look at her eyes and I see her fight back tears.

"Hello."

"Now I understand they have you all shook up today. We just need to do a quick x-ray of your chest."

"Can Matt…"

"Of course, Matt will be right here. Now let's get you out of that bed." Matt and Marg transfer me out of my bed. They help me towards a chair to sit in. I sit down, trembling, sweating, afraid.

Marg hands Matt a lead jacket and thyroid cover. I see him expertly get himself dressed in the items. This is his work life, I remind myself; he does this every day.

I sure don't.

Through the entire x-ray process, I can see Matthew from my vantage point. He checks the quality of the images with Marg and they announce that we are done. Matt scoops me up single-handedly and places me back on the bed. I see Marg's eyes not be able to contain her tears.

"Okay, now. Let us get you a warm blanket. You are freezing, my dear." My teeth are chattering and I cannot stop shaking. I see Marg hug Matthew and pat his shoulder. I see his shoulders lower and relax into her touch. They wrap me up in a fresh, warm blanket, and we return to the patient waiting area for the orderly to come and get me again.

Lying on the bed and waiting for the orderly to return, I am in full shock. My body is shaking uncontrollably and I want to vomit. Matt rushes over to me. He climbs onto the bed and wraps his arms around me and starts to rub my arms and legs furiously.

"Breathe, gumdrop. Breathe."

I am crying uncontrollably. This has all been too much. Too chaotic. Fear rips down my body.

"You are shocky. What can I do? What do you need?"

"Touch my face. Matt, touch my face."

With a concerned face, he takes his hands on either side of my face. I instantly relax into his warm hands. He takes his fingers and runs them gently down the bridge of my nose. I melt into his touch. This is what I needed.

"You are getting some color back."

"Do that again."

"I did this all the time when you were asleep."

"It relaxes me."

I see a smirk cross his lips. We share a small smile. I put my head on his shoulder and begin to be able to feel more like myself again. The orderly comes around the corner and scowls at Matt sitting in the bed with me.

"Those things aren't designed for that kind of weight," he grumps at us.

Matt ignores him entirely and gets off the bed. He holds my hand as we are wheeled back upstairs to my room. Getting off the elevator, I no longer hear the woman screeching down the hall. I am relieved. And suddenly, very hungry.

They wheel me back into my room and I see it filled with sunshine. My breakfast with real food has been dropped off as well. I am excited to see the prospect of actual solid food for the first time in a week.

They transfer me back to my own bed. The nurse comes in and says the doctor has said it is time to take out my catheter. I want to jump for joy. I ask her if I can eat a little first, and she obliges and says she will be back in a moment.

Matthew is already putting some peanut butter on my toast for me and cracking into the juice.

"Here, drink this," he says firmly, handing me the apple juice. "It will help the shock."

"I am feeling much better, love."

"I know. Drink your juice." His tone is nonnegotiable. I have scared him. I instantly feel bad.

I begin to eat my breakfast, which by now, is more like brunch. It is cold, but tastes good nonetheless. I can find my breath again and I glance around our room. Our little room is in shambles. The constant in and out of people, Matt's suitcase, which he can only throw things into before running to the next test, or my next request, is open and strewn about. There are stacks of magazines and cords from Matt's work laptop hanging around. I sit there and realize the chaos we are in. Chaos will not help us heal. Matt sees me staring at it all and reads my mind. He gets up from his breakfast and begins to pick things up a bit.

Just then, the phone rings. Matt answers it

"Yes, you can send her down... Thank you."

"What is it, hun?" I look down at my hospital gown. I am half-covered in crumbs and completely dishevelled.

"It is Jane. She is here."

Jane! My darling Jane. Jane, our dear friend, oh and I am a mess. Half-ashamed of the mess I am in, yet so relieved to see a real woman, one of my women. I want to get out of the bed and run into her arms.

She knocks and comes into the doorway. The instant I lay eyes on her, she wells with tears. She is instantly protesting;

"I do not want to intrude. I just wanted to drop these off." She is holding the most beautiful bouquet of white flowers. "Please, I am sorry..."

I see the stroller handle behind her. She has baby Anne with her. Oh my sweet baby, Anne.

"Please, no! Do not protest. My love. I am sorry I am such a mess." We both are teary, afraid to say the truth.

"It's just ... I was so scared ... " I could hear her palpable fear. She thought she was going to lose me. My heart broke wide open. "And the baby ..." her voice trailing off.

Just then, Anne fussed in stroller. I saw Jane glance heavily at me, wondering what to do.

"It is okay. Anne, sweetie, let me see her."

"Are you sure it is okay?"

"Of course it is." I sit further up in my bed and attempt to tidy myself. Jane bends down and gets 9-month-old Anne from her stroller and holds her in her arms. She smiles at me. I do the same. I cannot go to her, as I am chained down with my catheter and IV, but I wave and smile from my bed.

Jane stays a few moments. We don't address the elephant in the room. I tell her the doctors are happy with my progress and we promise to let her know what is going on. She takes her leave with wee Anne. Matt puts the flowers on the window sill.

I lay back and, for the first time, I understand why people bring flowers. They are something happy to look at. Spending more time awake now, with the narcotics wearing off, I can feel the grief creeping in. My mind overflows with questions. How did this happen? We just had her baby shower! I am seething in anger when my nurse, Daria, comes in to remove my catheter.

I must have turned pale as she approached the bed, as Matthew was suddenly at my side. Daria went to lift the blanket and I felt bile rise in my throat.

"The last nurse. She hurt me." My voice is barely audible.

Daria looks shocked. "Well, I will not hurt you. This process shouldn't hurt. All I am doing is removing the water from the tube that is holding the catheter in place. Then the catheter should just slip out."

"Are you sure?" I just don't know if I can trust her not to hurt me.

"Yes. I will go slowly and you can just talk to me."

I look up at Matt, who is standing at my bedside. His eyes are assuring me that everything will be okay. I relent.

The procedure is quick, although Daria brings in two students and has to teach them how to complete it, so it takes longer for her explanations. I am lying half-naked from the waist and being stared at by three women as they work on taking out my catheter. It is humbling and exhausting. It does not hurt. Only a slight tug and the damned catheter is out. I am instantly relieved and can sit with much more comfort.

Daria and her compliment of nurses leave and our room falls silent. For the first time since first thing this morning, our room falls quiet. Matt and I side glance at one another. Matt flops down on his cot, which creaks under his weight.

"This thing is so uncomfortable."

"Trade ya?"

He looks up at me and smirks.

"Nah. I still have the better deal."

He lies back and stares at the shelf above his cot. I follow his line of sight to the white box above him on the shelf.

"Matt?"

Grunts.

"What is in the box?"

I see him freeze. He holds his breath a moment.

"Things. Things of the baby's. The nurses gave it to me."

"What sort of things?"

"I do not know."

"You have not looked at it?"

"No. I couldn't." His voice is filled with resignation. "Dad took photos of her. I have them here, on the laptop," he says, pointing to his night bag at the foot of his bed.

"Oh." I am not sure what to think. I want to see her again. I am curious. But what is in those photos? Will it be gruesome? I could not stand it if she looks a mess. Lost in my own thoughts, I look up to see Matt's eyes on mine.

"Do you want to see her photos? She looks... different than when you saw her."

"Different? Different how?"

"Her lips. They are dark. And you are in the photos too. The nurse took a photo with you, and me, and the baby."

Dark lips? My stomach flips. I do not want to see death on my baby. I am afraid, and my hands are shaking.

"I want to see her."

Matt reaches down into his night bag and picks out the laptop. He places the five-pound netbook into my outstretched hand. The laptop is light. Matt bought it for me last Christmas with the intention that it would be my computer to use instead of the desktop with the baby. White and "chicky," as he put it, it was my treasure and I adored it. The second he places it in my hand, it feels like a 50-pound weight in my hand. My arm falls under its weight and Matt catches it.

"Easy there!" he chuckles.

"Did the laptop just kick my ass?" I am laughing. "I am so weak. I tried to hold onto it but couldn't."

"Here." Matt wheels over my meal tray and places it on top of it. "Let this do the work for you."

Matt goes over and lays down on his cot and closes his eyes. I stare at the home screen, willing myself to have the courage to open the link.

I cannot.

I cannot open the link. I close my eyes and rest back on the pillow behind me.

"We are going to be so screwed up, for so long, Matt."

He sighs deeply. "I know."

"How did we get here?"

"I do not know," he replies softly.

Tears choke at the back of my throat. "We are going to need counselling, Matt. We may need to see Kathy."

I wait. Kathy was a therapist we saw years before. Matt wasn't a huge fan of spending money on counselling. Holding my breath, I wait for his response.

"I was thinking that too."

I see a tear fall down the corner of his eye on the pillow he is laying on. They match the ones on my cheeks.

"Oh. We are so fucked up."

I stare at the computer screen in front of me. I move the mouse curser over the photos folder marked "Baby Krawecki" right in the middle of the desktop. Just as I do, there is a loud knock on our door. Startled, I jump and quickly slam shut the laptop, my quiet moment of courage squelched. In walks the resident doctor once again. His throng of followers is with him. He walks up to the foot of my bed and Matt stands up.

"She has no fluid in her lungs. They are clear. There is no need for further testing."

I see Matt take a deep breath, which is followed quickly by a look of regret. He feels badly for this morning. I can see it on his face. Poor guy. I reach out and take his hand.

"Thank you," I say warmly. The throng leaves with no further comment. The tall, lanky, young doctor looks back and smiles.

His face is warm and I wonder if he would have handled this all a little differently.

The moment the door latches shut, Matt turns to me,

"I am so sorry, babe. They said there was fluid. I thought you could have pneumonia."

"Don't apologize for taking care of me."

He sits down hard on the bed. He looks weary. His phone vibrates on the nightstand.

"Who is that?"

"Everyone."

I shoot him a quizzical look.

"Everyone. Caroline, Jen, Jade, Kath, looking for updates."

"You should get out of here a while. Get some fresh air. A shower. A shave."

"I will rest when you rest." He lies back on the cot and closes his eyes.

The same answer I always get. My loyal husband, never leaving my side.

We spend an hour or two napping and resting. The narcotics are slowly wearing off and I am slowly being freed of this medical prison inside my head. My mom calls the room and says she is coming by later after supper. Hearing that Mom is coming, Matthew finally agrees to take leave for a bit and to go out and get some fresh air. He kisses my forehead and I assure him I will be okay until he comes back.

The orderly comes by with my supper. Some sort of stew, the obligatory cheese and crackers, juice, and ginger ale. I look at it. It does not smell right. This hospital food is beginning to be as foul as this place I am in. I push my tray aside and decide to walk to the bathroom to freshen myself up. I swing my legs over the side of the bed and bear my weight upon them. I hang onto the side of the bed and find that I am okay. I can stand. I stand up a little further and feel my staples pull along my ribcage.

"Ouch!" I put my hand over my right rib. It feels tender, sore. The painkillers are letting go and the pain is increasing just as they said it would. I feel anger build in my belly.

"Screw this," I mutter. I shuffle my body away from the bed, determined to make the 10 feet to the bathroom. I keep one hand steady on the wall. The weight of my empty belly hangs as I am half-hunched over, unable to stand up erect. I shuffle-step my way to the bathroom and sit down on the toilet with a thump.

I made it. A small victory.

I shuffle-step back out into the hallway towards the bathroom sink. Hunched over, I wash my hands. My nails are filthy. When is the last time anyone helped me wash myself? I need a shower. I doubt they will let me. I scrub my hands until they are mine again. I see beside the sink that Matt has brought me my make-up case and travel bag. I open it and find nail clippers; a small token to help humanize me. On the counter, is a bag of nightgowns my sister and

Dad brought for me. I eagerly get out of my hospital gown and put on the soft cotton gown. My clever sister included a scarf that I can throw over my shoulder to keep warm. I am grateful. Feeling a bit better and more myself, I am about to head back to bed when I catch my reflection in the mirror.

My eyes are large. Wide. My face nearly gaunt. I was a plump-and-happy pregnant lady, full cheeked and lipped from the greatness of pregnancy, and now I am drawn. My face is sharp-featured. Where did all my weight go? I must be 20 pounds lighter in just a week. On the side of my neck is a big, black, stitch. The central line they took out. I run my hand over it. It is painful and dark.

"That will scar," I mutter. A quarter-inch scar to carry on my neck for the rest of my life.

My neck and collar bones jut out. My hair, wild and untamed. I go through the make-up kit and find hair elastics and clips to hold it down. My legs are beginning to wobble, and I know I must head back to bed soon. I steady myself by hanging onto the counter and shuffle my way back to bed.

I pass by the window. It's growing dark outside. Another night is coming. Another horrid night. I sit down on the bed and lift my legs one-by-one back in. The gown is soft and the scarf helps me feel more covered up. I glance over at the food and figure I should try and eat. I need out of this hospital and eventually, they are going to care if I eat.

I pick and putter at the food. It is too salty and rich. The juice and crackers go down well and I set extras aside. We are beginning to hoard good snack food Matt and I have to have between meals.

Just then, there is a light knock on the door.

A warm face comes around the corner. It is my Tante Linda.

Carrying a small potted marigold plant, her smile is as wide as her face.

"Hello, Peanut," she says.

Peanut. Peanut, because once when I was 3, I shoved a peanut, without its shell, up my nose when she was babysitting me. She had to figure out how to get it out with a pair of tweezers before my mother came and picked me up. This peanut will never live it down, from the peanut-themed wedding gift to my nickname. I adore her and the loving tease of peanut. I am relieved to see her. In fact, I can barely remember when the last time was. Perhaps a couple years before, at our wedding. Seeing her standing at the foot of my bed drives home just how bad this is. I hear her condolences. Her wet eyes tell me just how sad she is that we lost our daughter. Tante Linda is my mom's best friend. She would come when things were bad. Through the lifting medicine fog, I am slowly coming to realize just how close to death I was. Somehow, ever since I woke up, I have been in survival mode. And now I see that I almost died. My baby died. My baby with no name.

Tante Linda stays a short while and makes me laugh with her humor about the bad hospital food. Her company is warm and lovely. She takes her leave as I am beginning to tire and she can see it.

I push my hospital tray away and decide to close my eyes a while. I drift into sleep gently, when I hear a man clear his throat at the end of the bed. I open my eyes and *it is him.*

Dr. Dewitt. Mr. "Your baby has expired."

Adrenaline races through my body. What is he doing there? Am I awake? Am I dreaming? He does not work at this hospital. Hasn't he done enough? I am paralyzed with fear.

"How are you doing?" he asks, taking no pause for my answer. "I thought I would come in and see you..."

His mouth is moving, but I cannot hear his voice. All I can hear is the blood rushing in my ears. I am terrified. Alone. Very much awake. Shaking, I look over at the call button. It is too obvious. I cannot hit it without him seeing.

"I hear that Dr. McMillan was able to save your uterus. That is good..."

He is still talking? Does he not see the sweat across my lip? I am having a full panic attack by his very presence and he is talking to me about my uterus.

"I am sorry, Dr. Dewitt," I stammer, "I am still recovering..."

"Yes, I would be happy to see you after your recovery here so we can discuss your options."

"My options? What options?"

"Well yes, as you recover, I am sure you will want a lot of answers. I can help you with those." He stands up straighter "Although, I should say, it is unclear as to whether you will be able to have any more children."

The room spins. Bile rises in my throat. I am gripped in fear. More children? I can't have more children? But I want my daughter! I want to be a Mom! Is he saying I will never be a Mom? I had never thought that all this meant I would never be a Mom. I do not even know what this means.

"Please. Dr. Dewitt. I am very tired."

"Of course. I will leave my contact information at the desk and you can come and see me when you are ready."

He leaves and I curl up and hyperventilate into my pillow. Crawled onto my side and curled up in a ball, I hyperventilate, gripping into the bed in fear. I can't have more children? Did they sterilize me? What happened to me? What was this disease? I want my baby back! Does this mean no more children, ever? I sob and shake. On a rotating carousel of nightmare, I never know what will come at the next knock of the door. My dear, sweet Tante Linda was just here and now this? Chaos. Through my sobs and screams, I do not even hear my mother come in.

She finds me shaking and curled up on my side in bed.

"Oh, sweetheart. Sweetheart!" Her voice brings me back to reality. I fall into her lap like a child and sob. She runs her hand over my head and tries to soothe me. "Tell me."

"The doctor. The doctor."

"Which doctor?"

"Dewitt. He said I cannot have any more kids. He said, he wasn't sure. Mom! What did they do to me?"

Her blue eyes blaze. She sits up and grabs me hard by the shoulders. "Now you listen to me. Look at me when I say this; Matthew and I talked to Dr. McMillan. We talked to him. He said it was still an option. He said. And he was the one that operated on you. This Dewitt guy, he doesn't know."

I crumble into tears and let it all pour out. The chaos and the heartache. I sob in her lap like a child. Completely undone.

When Matthew returns a short time later, I have collected myself and washed my face. My Mom pulls him into the hallway to talk, but I can feel his anger when he walks into the room. He comes over and strokes the bridge of my nose gently before settling into his cot. We say nothing. Nothing needs to be said.

That night, I am lying in bed, watching the snowflakes fall outside our 7th-story window. Matt is there, watching "Mr. Sunshine," a bad Matthew Perry show that lasted only a few episodes before mercifully being taken off the air. Our visitors are gone for the day, and the hospital is quiet and most patients are in their rooms.

An orderly comes in and gives us a "Valentine's Day treat," a two-bite brownie with a pink frosting heart on top. I count on my fingers; I guess it is Valentine's Day. The days are blurring together.

Matt stares at it a while grumbling, "Well, that will ruin two-bite brownies for me for the rest of my life."

I can't care about the brownie, which he is now happily devouring. I am SO uncomfortable. My staples are pulling and I keep sliding down in the bed. This ward bed must have been made in 1929 because it is digging into my back and I can't get comfortable.

Strapped to the bed, my catheter pulls with every shift I make. My IV line snakes all over my lap and I feel tangled in tubes and wires. Ugh. So uncomfortable.

"Matt, I can't get comfy."

He looks at me, half-heartedly, and says, "Put the head of the bed up more. Sitting up will put less pressure on the staples."

I raise the head of the bed and promptly slide down further; the slick plastic of the mattress interacting with the fabric of my nightgown and I am now one third of the way down the bed.

"Ugh, Matthew. This isn't working." I am peeking over the top of my blankets like a child in an oversized snowsuit.

Matt begins to chuckle. "You look like the bed ate you! Come here." He yanks on my arms to pull me up.

As soon as he lets go, I slide back down. The blankets are up in front of my face and I am seriously becoming frustrated.

"Matt!"

"Okay, that's it," I hear Matt say.

Suddenly, he climbs into the bed and straddles me. He wraps both arms around my waist and pulls me up in the bed. It works! I am sitting higher up and I feel the pressure come off my staples. But then it occurs to me; he is straddling me, on a bed, on Valentine's Day and I am just out of the ICU. This looks BAD.

"Matt, stop! Stop, Matt! Please! What if the nurse comes in! Matt!"

"Well, how else am I supposed to lift you? You keep sliding down! Besides, baby... it is Valentine's Day," he says with a growl, his face in mine.

I remember laughing in that moment like I had never laughed before. I remember tears rolling down our cheeks as he hurriedly got me into place and then jumped off the bed before we were busted like a pair of hormonal teenagers. I remember the fact that he smelt like brownie and the light I saw in his eyes for the first time in what seemed like forever. It was only six days after she died and still one of the funniest moments of my life.

The evening was winding down, and our lights dimmed. Matthew was changed into his PJs for yet another night at my hospital bedside. The hallways were as quiet as they were the night before when we were wheeled down. I was quietly looking out the window, thinking of our daughter, when there was a quiet knock on the door.

"Come in."

In walked Dr. Hernandez. I was shocked. It had to be almost bedtime. What was he still doing here? He looked tired. In his scrubs, he came in alone, with none of his straggling students behind him.

"Hello," he said, his soft accent a welcome air to the room. "I wanted update you."

"Dr. Hernandez, you must be exhausted!"

His eyes sparkled and a familiar smirk returned to his lips. He pauses and observes me before replying. "You look different to me." He glanced at Matt. "Doesn't she look different?"

Matt smiled in return. "This is her."

"Very different from when we met, no?"

"Yes. She did not look like herself when you met her. This is my girl."

I sat between them, wondering just how bad things were when I was asleep. Sitting here, my hair tamed, in a fresh gown and scarf. This *is* me. Who was I before?

"Well, I have good news. Your liver enzymes are continuing to come back down. It will take time. We need to do a CT scan of the liver to ensure that all is healing well."

I feel adrenaline course through me. Another CT scan? Panicking, I glance at Matt. But the last one, it was so bad.

"Will dye be required?" Matthew's wits are sharp, even in pajama pants.

"Yes. We will need her to drink the dye solution. And have the injectable in through her IV."

I sit party to this conversation, as Matt advocates on my behalf. Terrified. More tests? Why can't they just leave me alone?

"Once we have the results from this CT scan, we can ensure her safety and that all is healing. Okay?" He smiles at me while I panic on the inside. I am not okay with more testing. I am not okay. "I will come back and check on you tomorrow. My resident will be checking in with you in the morning. We want to see that you are healing well before going any further."

I see Matthew's chest fall. That resident is not his first choice for my care. But being that Dr. Hernandez is in charge, there is little he can do.

"Thank you, Doctor."

"Yes, thank you," Matt said, grabbing my hand.

His calm, assuring energy should be enough to squelch my fears, but all I heard was that I need to have a CT, and by the sounds of things, I am never being released from this jail. I curl up on my side and cry. Matt, used to my tears by now, pats my hand and quietly says, "You can do the CT. I will be there."

We turn out the light and try to rest. It has been an exhausting day. The hospital days are filled with people, this rotating door in and out of constant activity with no privacy whatsoever. It leaves me drained and frustrated. Even as I try to drift off to sleep, I hear a nurse come in and poke her head around the corner to check on me. I find myself filled with anger; please, just leave me alone!

I toss and turn the first half of the night. My dreams are vivid and chaotic. No spiders or monsters, no death as the narcotics are coming out of my system, but I wake up confused, not knowing where I am. Somewhere in the night, the nurse comes by to take my vitals. She mentions that my temperature is high and that she needs to take my blood pressure. It is on the high side of normal. I drift in and out, wanting peace and relief and finding none.

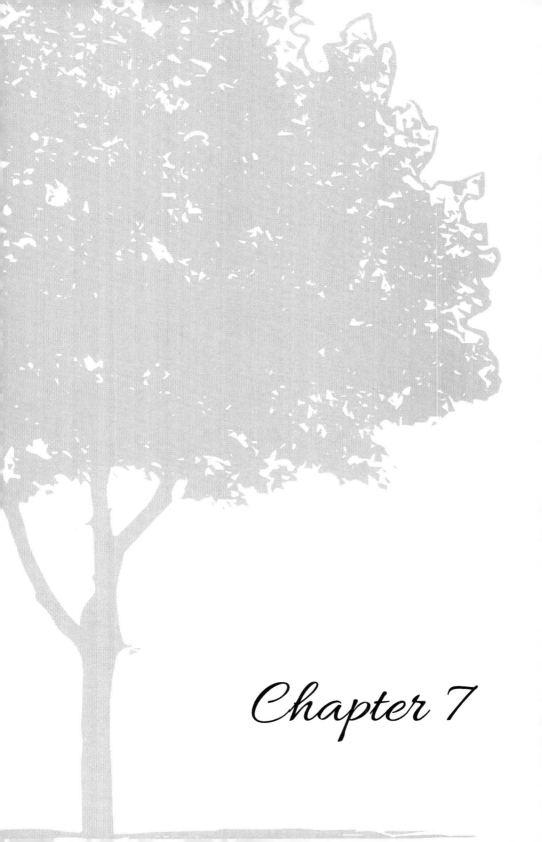

Chapter 7

Tuesday

Our Tuesday morning wake-up call comes identical to Monday's.

Slam! Bang!

The orderly comes in and removes the laundry bag from the night before. She lets the lid fall onto the empty basket and it rings noise into the room. Matt angrily rolls over and puts the pillow on his head.

"No decency!" he mutters in frustration.

Isn't that just the understatement of the century?

Remembering what happened the morning before, I get up and shuffle my way to the bathroom. The resident and his minions will arrive with his orders. I want to be ready. Please, let Tuesday be kinder. Please.

As I brush my teeth and wet down my hair, I hear the door open. I am stricken with panic. Who is this now?

"Hello! Breakfast time." The orderly comes in with my breakfast tray. As she bangs into my room, I am badly startled. My heart is beating through my chest so fast, I can see it through my gown. I taste metal. I am half-panicked. I feel every cell in my being panic from having her enter the room. "This is not okay," is all I can think. "What is wrong with me? It is just breakfast!"

"Thanks. You can put it over there," I say, motioning to the tray table.

She leaves after depositing my breakfast and I stand, gripping the counter. *Breathe, Melissa, breathe. In. Out. In. Out.* This place has me rattled. That revolving door, I never know who is coming and when they are. I feel exposed and afraid here.

I shuffle back to bed and Matt sits up, smilingly warmly at me.

"Hey, look at you! You are walking around!"

"I still can't stand up straight," I said, still bent at the waist on an angle. "But I can move, so that is something."

"More than something, babe." His eyes are warm and kind.

I sit on the bed and do not even have a moment to swing my legs onto the bed before there is another bang at the door as Mr. Resident and his team of shadows come into the room.

Only this time, Dr. Hernandez is with them, looking fresh-eyed and smiling. He must have fallen into a cot somewhere and slept, just to return first thing this morning. I am suddenly humbled.

The resident begins his usual routine where he prattles off my condition, while looking down at the charts and not making eye contact with me. I chuckle at the oddity of having your existence reduced to numbers and readings. Matt and I exchange an amused look. I notice Dr. Hernandez is paying no mind of the resident and rather, is watching me. As soon he is done, Dr. Hernandez interjects in.

"So we will order your CT today and we will get an idea from there, as we discussed last night."

I smirk and feel the bravery build in my belly.

"Today is Tuesday. The 15th."

"Yes it is." Dr. Hernandez looks down at my file.

"And my birthday is Friday the 18th. I need to be home for Friday. I need home to get better."

"Well, we need to..."

I stopped listening. I grin and sit back. Point made. I am going home Thursday, even if I have to sign myself out of this insane place. I see from the look in Matthew's eyes that he can tell what I am thinking,

"You are trouble," he murmurs as the hoard of doctors ignore us at the foot of the bed. "You will have to walk out over my dead body..."

"That can be arranged." I smile back at him. He shakes his head with a chortle in his throat.

The doctors leave with little fanfare. Matt and I split the gigantic breakfast they have sent me and we begin to settle into the day. I somehow manage to convince Matt to go back to my parents' house and try to get some time away from this place. The CT will not be until later in the day by the time they get everything arranged. He begrudgingly agrees. I know he needs a nap and a hot shower. I feel the need to be alone, and between the nurses and his prying blue eyes, I barely have a moment to myself. He steps out, promising to come straight back and asks that I call him if I need anything.

I can hear voices in the hall and commotion up and down. This floor is noisy. I thought it was quiet, thanks to the noise of the ICU, but perspective tells me different. With Matthew gone and finally all by myself, I begin to move around the room. Picking up and folding laundry. Putting away clutter. These rooms are tiny and we are practically living on top of each other. I have to move very slowly. Each raise of my arms is effort. Each turn pulls and tugs at my incisions. I move with great deliberation.

"Jesus," I mutter. "I am so weak."

My belly aches. I put my hand underneath it to support its weight as I walk. My stomach is so still. She is dead. My eyes sting hotly. She is still dead. How can this be?

I see the laptop Matthew left out at the foot of the bed. I pick it up and sit down on the edge of the bed. It is time to see her. Just me and her.

I open the laptop and sink back into the bed. I pray no one comes in and interrupts this moment. Matthew has left the folder right in the middle of the desktop. It is labeled "Baby Krawecki."

Baby.

She does not have a name. I am not sure I want to name her. I do not want to believe she is dead. I want a redo. I do not want to name a baby I do not get to bring home. I love all the names we picked out so much. If I use one of them, then it is real. Our baby is dead.

I take a deep breath and click the link. Instantly, she is up on the screen. Wrapped in her pink blanket. My eyes instantly fall on her black lips. Her lips did not look like that when I met her. I can see the marks of death on her face. Greys and blues with black lips. I can barely stand to look.

No. No. Hot tears pour down my cheeks. This isn't how she was! She was pink and perfect and cold, but not like this. I click through the photos and see how my family took pictures of all of her. Her hands, her feet. Her cute little hat and the swooped bridge of her nose.

Like mine.

I find myself reaching out and touching the screen, as if to touch her face. There are photos of each person in my family holding her, except my father, who was taking the pictures. As I scroll through, attempting to absorb the moment they were in, I come to a photo of Matthew and his girl. Just the two of them curled up on the sofa, her resting in the crook of his arm.

He is a Dad. My Matthew is a Dad. He looks so natural there with her. I always knew he would be a good Dad, and there he is. And I didn't get to see it. He looks so in love and I never got to see him fall in love with his baby.

I click the next picture and see my brother is beside Matthew now. His body language is strong. He is reserved. His hands clasped, his shoulders down and back and he sits beside Matthew. I can tell he is holding back. I can tell he is holding space. And then in a click of the mouse, I see him holding her.

And I gasp.

The love I see on his face for my girl leaps off the screen and hits me square in the chest with a crushing weight. He loves her. She is his. I can see through his face and eyes that she is his, and he wanted her just as we did.

She must be Ava.

My Ava. She is Ava. I take a deep breath with her for a moment. *My Ava.*

Suddenly, there is a knock on the door and I close the laptop quickly.

"Hello, hello," a soft voice comes from around the corner. It is my Dad.

"Hey, Dad." Our eyes meet and a soft smile is exchanged. I can see his eyes are tired.

"How is today?" he asks, as he takes off his jacket and sits in the chair at the foot of my bed.

"Okay. Apparently, they are sending me for a CT soon. Depending on those results, they may send me home."

He nods.

"I see you have lunch there," he motions at the tray across the room from me. "Let me bring that over for you."

Dad and his kids and food.

I lift up the cover to see the same supper as last night: dodgy, thick, slimy, and over-salted beef stew. With it, they have generously included a bun, crackers, a fruit cup, cheese, and a rice pudding dessert. My appetite is less than nil, but I want out of this bed, and I know choking down this food may help me get stronger. I push the stew around my bowl and pick out all of the vegetables to eat.

"Need a hand with that?" Dad says with a smirk. "You know, you actually have to eat it, to eat it."

"Carrots don't come in this shape," I retort, holding up a preformed "carrot" cube. "Last time I checked, anyways."

"You love rice pudding. Look! Rice pudding. That looks good!" I can see him smile as he attempts to cheer me on. "Here, let me open that for you." He is right, I do love rice pudding; his rice pudding. My Nana's recipe that is cooked long and sweetly on the stove; it is soft, with just the right amount of sweetness. I take a look into the pudding to see a congealed, cold, and tough slop.

"This is not rice pudding, Dad."

"What do you mean? Yes, it is."

Picking it up, I turn it completely upside down. I shake it, for emphasis, "rice pudding. Does. Not. Do. This." It remains in its container, as my eyes are fixed on his. Just then, I see his façade fold and we dissolve in tears of laughter.

Just then, there is a second knock at the door. My nurse walks in and she is carrying a huge jug of what appears to be water, and a small Styrofoam cup.

"Hey, Melissa. I am sorry to do this but we have to send you for a CT in 45 minutes. I need you to drink this entire jug," she sets it down on my bed tray, "in that time."

"You need me to drink over a litre of THAT in 45 minutes?" My eyes widen and I glance at my father. He shakes his head and his arms cross. This is ridiculous.

"Normally, we would be able to give you two hours to do so, but we have had a scheduling change." She gives me a sympathetic look as she pours me a cup of it and hands it to me. "It just tastes like salty water. It allows them to get a better picture."

"This is insane," I hear my Dad mutter from behind her.

I take the cup and stare at it. Time is wasting, so I take a sip and feel gross as I do so. It is like salted water, only somehow oily. I cannot fathom finishing the glass, never mind that entire jug. I feel as if I have been tested with eating a mountain. The nurse quietly scurries out of the room and I sigh.

"This place is ridiculous. I cannot even lift the jug to refill it, yet I am supposed to drink all this?"

"In 40 minutes," Dad grumbles, checking his watch. He comes over and refills my cup. I can see his frustration. I feel trapped, but I need this CT, and if this is when I have do to it, what choice do I have? I gulp down the disgusting solution and stare at the jug. Barely a dent made and the clock continues to tick.

Dad and I sit in silence, me drinking, him refilling for some time. A second nurse comes in.

"Hallo, my dear. I just need to start your IV antibiotics."

"I am trying to drink this," I say, pointing to the gigantic one litre jug of fluid in front of me. "Is there any way this could wait?"

"Oh, you will have some time. When are they sending you for the test?"

"Twenty minutes," my father responds from behind her.

"Twenty minutes! And they just gave you this now?" she asks, pointing to the jug.

"Yes. This isn't going to happen, is it?"

Her eyebrows raise and her face says that I am right; this isn't going to happen. I glance at the jug; it is almost half-way gone. The nurse leaves, saying she will be back to start my IV, and Dad and I stare at the jug once more.

"Fuck it." Anger seers through me.

He nods in response and takes the jug away.

Sure enough, no one comes back in 20 minutes to take me down for the CT. Dad and I small talk about the hospital. He says that my sister is here with him, just in the waiting room.

"Can I see her?" I ask.

"Of course, Petunia. Let me get her for you." He comes over and kisses my forehead before leaving.

Kath comes into the room looking flustered. I can see the stress on her face and I want to reach across the room and pull her into the bed with me. I want us to curl up and watch *Little House on the Prairie,* the one where Mary goes blind and all feels lost. I want to eat junk food and hide under the blankets, and pretend we are back in bed and girls again. Instead, we small chat a while and I tell her about the ridiculousness that this morning has been.

"Where is Leo?" I ask.

Instantly, I see her eyes well with hot tears. She places her face in her hands and begins to tremble. I instantly regret the question and am flooded with compassion.

"He is down the hall. With Dad."

"Why?"

"Because!" I hear the anger bite the back of her throat. "Because it is not fair. I have him and you don't ... you don't ... and I want you to love him. But how can you? I have two and you have none."

She sits just outside my reach from the bed. I cannot get to her. I lean as far forward as I can and reach my entire body towards her.

"Sister. Sister, please. Kath. Sister." Her flashing green eyes meet mine. "Go get Leo. Go get him right now."

She looks shocked by my response. She shakes her head no and I nod mine in return.

"Bring him to me."

She leaves the room a moment and I sit back in bed and think. How do I do this? How? Before I have a chance to answer, I hear the door open and in she walks with him in her arms. I can see she is afraid to hurt me and she stands on guard to protect me. I look at him; he is big. Bigger than my Ava. Much bigger; a babe full-term, plus 6 weeks. Much bigger than my 5 pound, 10 ounce girl at 34+6. She sits across from me and I study his face. He isn't Ava.

"Can I hold him?"

She brings him over and places him in my arms. He is heavy. Far heavier than I can lift and I adjust my body so I can support his weight. I feel my staples pull and I ignore them. I take a deep breath and look down at his sweet face. His eyes meet mine and I am slammed, stunned, and speechless. He is perfect. Just like she was.

They are a pair.

They were together. Wherever they came from, they were together. He was the last person in our family that saw her, held her, and loved her before coming here. He knows her. They are bound together, somehow, unimaginably.

I lean down and kiss the top of his head and feel its warmth. But he isn't her. She was cold. And he is going to forever remind me of her and what she will not be. She will be his shadow in each and every way, only now, he will be what she does not get to be. I feel every cell in my body scream at the thought. Suddenly, in front of me, I see birthdays, Christmas, celebrations that she will not have. That I will watch him have, without her. My mind begins to spin and I scream for it to stop.

"I choose love," I say quietly only to Leo. He looks up at me and I see his soft eyes affirming my choice. I choose to love this little boy more fiercely, with a wild abandon and a conscious choice that I will be loving in this loss. This will not destroy us. I will not allow it.

I look up and see my sister's eyes and in it, the fear for the pain she is causing. She is not. She takes Leo from my arms and we chat as sisters do. And she leaves me to rest with a kiss.

Dad returns to my room and he offers to take me for a walk down the hall. Getting my housecoat on, I shuffle-step slowly beside him. He stands tall and firm while supporting my arm. I am humbled instantly. Here is my Dad, my childhood hero, walking me slow and steady down the hall. Wasn't I supposed to be taking care of him? I am filled with thoughts of how wrong this situation feels, yet I am comforted by his strength and determination to get me well. This is his way of loving me right now and I am grateful.

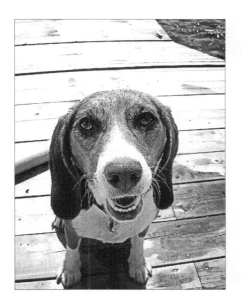

CHARLIE AKA THE BEAGS

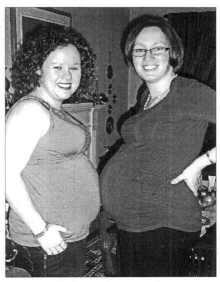

KATH AND I PREGNANT WITH AVA AND LEO ON CHRISTMAS 2010, THIS IS THE ONLY PHOTO WE HAVE OF THOSE TWO TOGETHER.

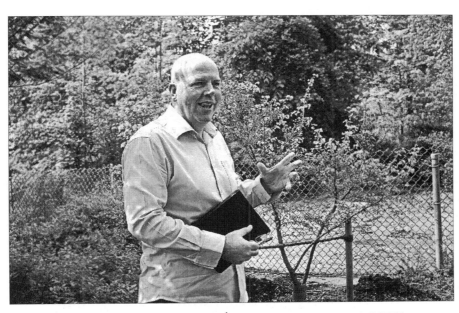

WAYNE PREVETT OFFICIATING AVA'S MEMORIAL SERVICE IN MAY 2011.

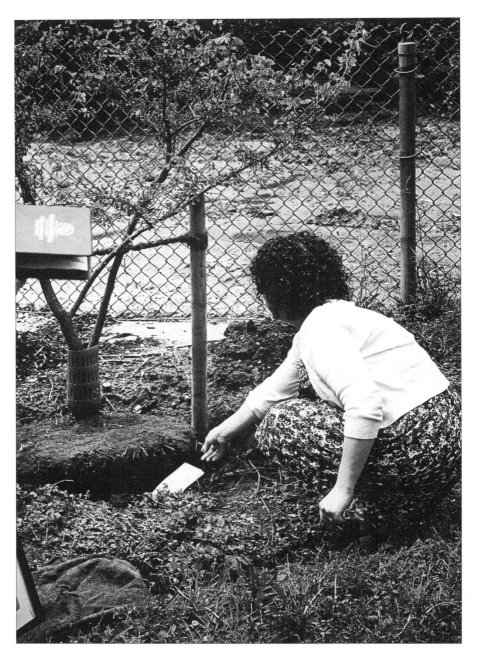

PLACING MY LETTER TO AVA WITH HER TREE,
A LETTER SOLELY BETWEEN HER AND I WHAT WAS
WRITTEN WILL ALWAYS BE IN MY HEART.

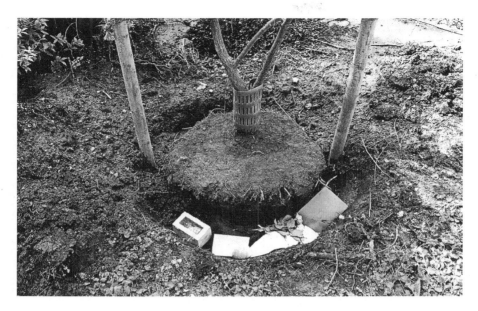

ITEMS WE PLACED WITH HER TREE

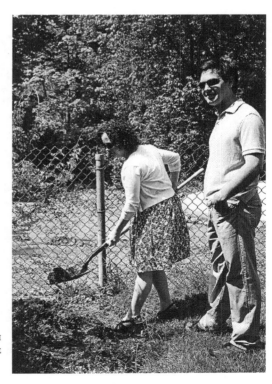

MATTHEW AND I
PLANTING HER TREE

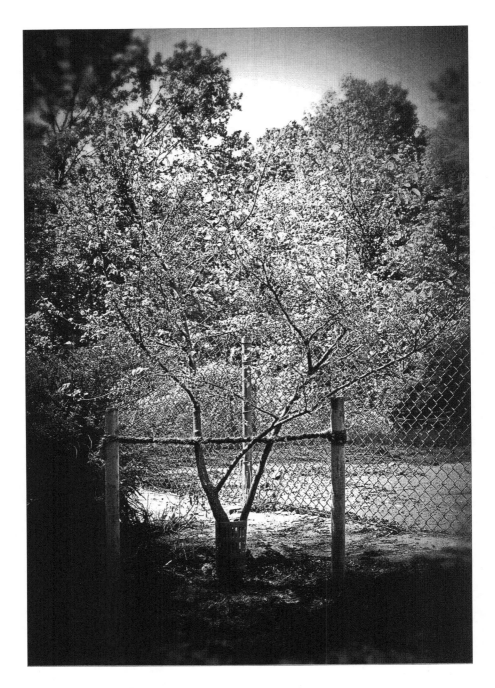

AVA'S TREE IN ALL ITS GLORY THE DAY WE PLANTED IT

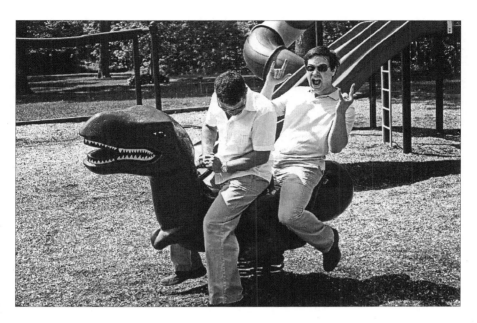

GUS AND MATT PLAYING AT THE PARK NEARBY.

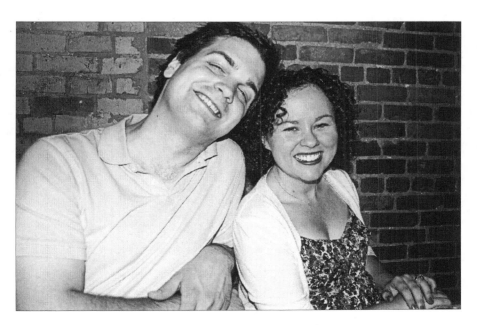

MATTHEW AND I AT AVA'S MEMORIAL LUNCH

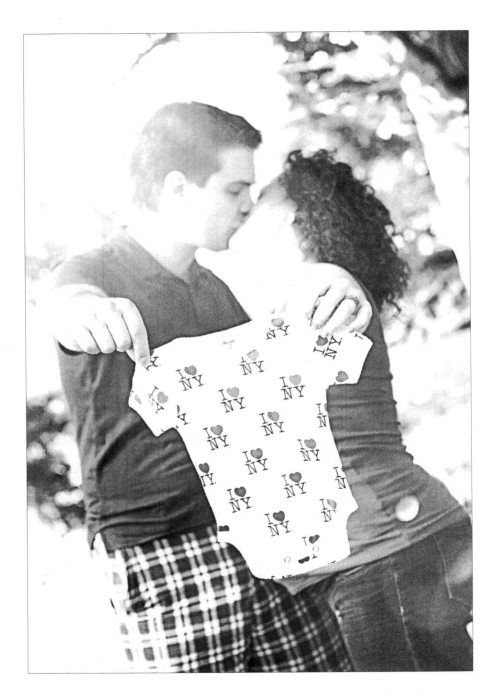

HARTISTREE PHOTOGRAPHICS AND A RAINBOW NYC ONESIE

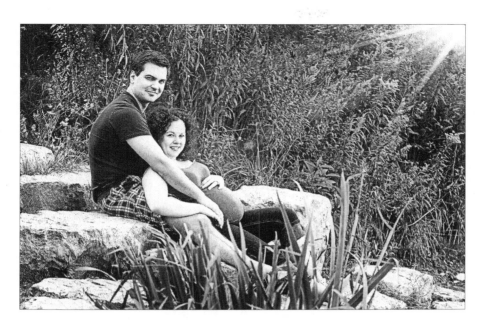

HARTISTREE PHOTOGRAPHICS

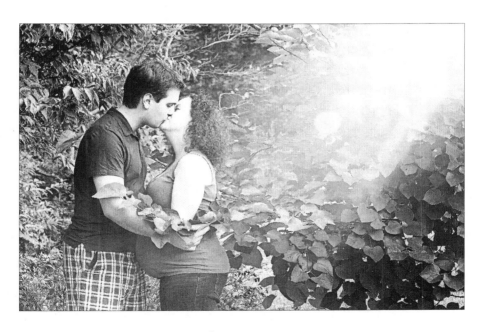

MATTHEW AND I WITH AVA'S TREE - HARTISTREE PHOTOGRAPHICS

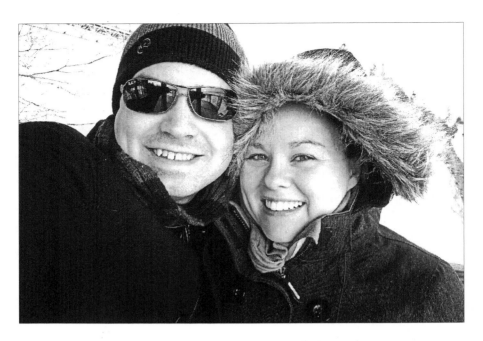

MATTHEW AND I IN QUEBEC CITY FOR AVA'S 1ST BIRTHDAY,
I FOUND OUT I WAS PREGNANT AGAIN TWO DAYS LATER

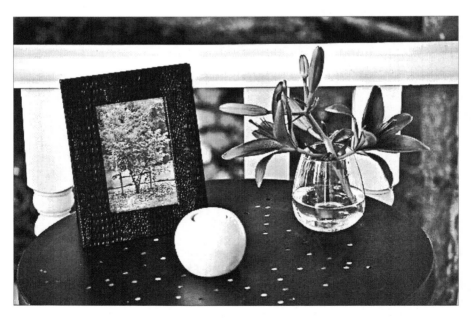

JANE INCLUDED AVA AT HER *HIGH TEA* TO CELEBRATE MY PREGNANCY

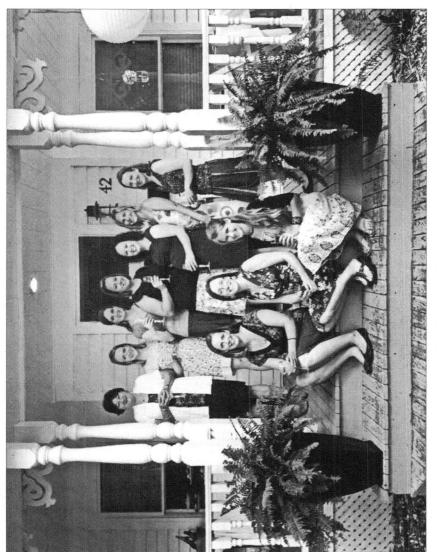

MY WOMEN CELEBRATING *HIGH TEA*

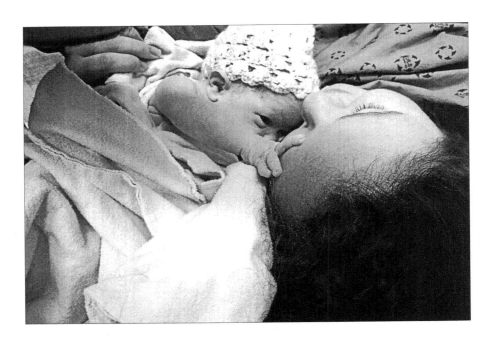

THE BEST MOMENT OF MY LIFE, MEETING LILLIAN

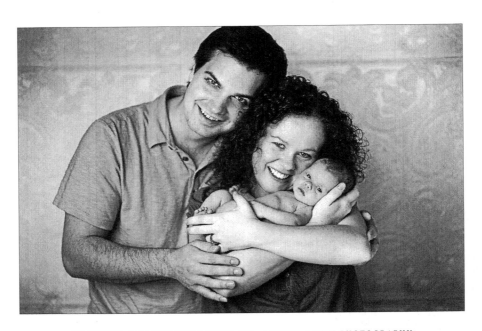

MATTHEW, LILLIAN AND I WITH AVA, ALWAYS - HRM PHOTOGRAPHY

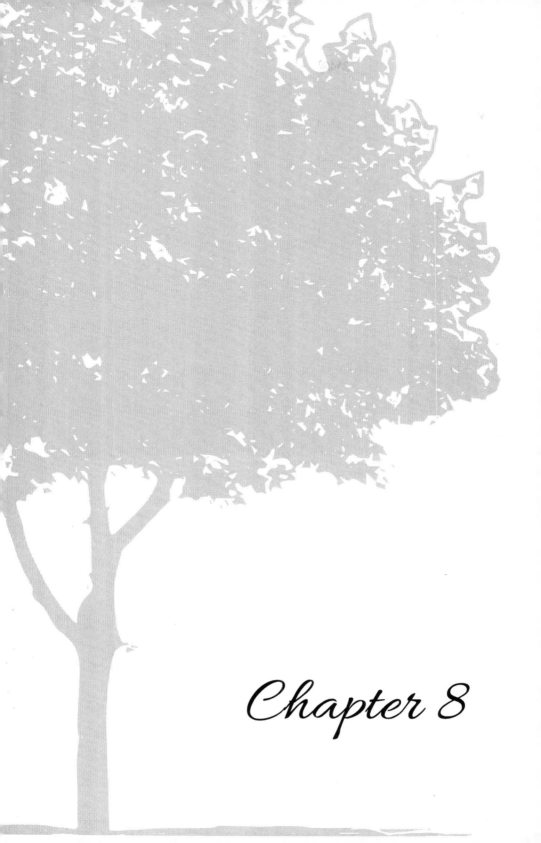

Chapter 8

Wednesday

The next morning, Dr. Hernandez comes into my room with a smile. He apologizes profusely for the confusion of the day before regarding the CT scan. He has scheduled a CT for that morning, with adequate time to drink the solution required, and says he will be back in later in the evening to discuss what they have seen.

"Friday is my birthday," I say, my voice small. "I really would like to be home for my birthday."

"What is the day today?" Dr. Hernandez asks, turning to his resident beside him.

"Wednesday."

A smile comes across his lips. "Well, let us see. Are you getting around?"

"Yes. I have been up and walking a bit."

"Sir," the tall-and-lanky doctor at the back pipes up. All this time, I have never heard him speak. "I have seen her walking around myself. And the nurses say she went for a walk yesterday with her Dad."

I plaster a smile on my face; I know I must play the game. Just please get me out of here so I can go home and grieve. I cannot grieve here. Let me be.

"Well, let us see what today's tests bring."

After returning to our room later that morning and completing all of Dr. Hernandez's testing, our room was filled with silence.

"I have paperwork I have to get you to sign," Matt said quietly. "I am sorry. I tried to avoid this. There was a mix-up and now I have to take the paperwork to the funeral home. I am sorry." His eyes were on his shoes.

"Why are you sorry?"

"Because. I never wanted you to have to see this paper. I have read it. That is bad enough."

"What is it?"

"Her death certificate."

Silence rang through the room. He went over to his bag and began to dig through it.

"Just don't look at it. Don't read it."

"But I am signing it. Aren't I supposed to have read it?"

"No. You do not want to read this. It is bad. I have read it enough for both of us. Don't even look, just sign where I show you."

"Don't look. Just sign?"

"Yes."

He placed the paper on top of the table and covered as much of the paper with his hand that he could. I picked up the pen and saw him pointing beside "Signature of mother."

I am a mother?

Mother? A mother without a baby?

I shook the thought out of my head and simply signed. Matthew quickly scooped up the paper and turned his back as he walked away with it.

"Thank you, babe," I said quietly.

"I am just going to run this where I need to. Will you be okay?"

"Oh, yeah. Think I will call my pedicurist and maybe get a massage."

"Very funny."

"Is there anything I can get you?"

Ava.

"Um. I think I need my girls. Can you rally the women?"

"Who do you need?"

"Jen, Caroline..."

"Consider it done."

After he had gone, I found myself sitting in the quiet of the day. Sore and sick of sitting in the bed, I glanced up and saw that white box Matthew had been carting around so carefully. That white box.

Getting up and walking slowly and hunched over to the shelf he had placed it on. Sitting down in the only chair we had in the room. Opening it carefully, I had no idea what to expect, and I boldly spent half an hour pouring over each and every item in the box. Footprints, handprints, her hand mold.

And the tears came crashing down.

My afternoon was filled with friends. True to his word, Matthew rallied the women in our life, and Jen arrived shortly thereafter. As well, his best man and my pseudo-brother Jordan came. The company was dizzying and difficult, but comforting all at the same time. Jen had Matthew come to her house and pack up a care package of homemade lasagne, magazines, drinks, and things to keep us distracted. Jen is a nurse and was the first to grasp the true danger of our circumstances. She entered my room with such grave appreciation, and I could feel her tremble from across the room.

I nearly died.

And she did die.

That afternoon also came with an unexpected delivery. One of the many knocks on the door was a hospital volunteer.

"E-greetings," she said, her tone flat as she set a stack of paper on my bed.

"Pardon me?"

"E-greetings," and she turned and left.

What on earth is she talking about? I picked up the stack of paper that had to be at least 70 pages thick. Bound together by an elastic band, I flattened them out and lifted the first one off of the pile.

"I am so sorry for you loss..."

And the second one.

"You are so very missed around the office. I do not know what to say..."

And the third one.

"Thinking of you in this difficult time..."

All my coworkers, my bosses, and colleagues had taken the time to send me e-greetings. I read through letter after letter after letter, tears pouring down my face. I was one of them. I am part of their team. Moved and speechless, I tied them back up and put them under my pillow, treasured.

When Matthew returned from Jen and Jamie's, the smell of homemade lasagne filled our little room. Matt curled up on my tiny bed with me, and we sat and ate. My hunger was slowly returning, and my strength was coming back more with each bite.

"Oh, yum. Real food."

"I know, right?" Matt said between bites.

"Food that actually tastes good." As we sat there stuffing our faces and feeling the most normal we had in ages, Dr. Hernandez came back in. He said that they had seen a couple of "bubbles" on the CT. That they could have been air bubbles from the surgery, but that they could be infection related. If they were infection, they would need to do another procedure, but that they needed to make sure. He wanted to run a blood test to look at my white cell count. If it was not elevated, they would assume they are air bubbles that will resolve.

"And if they are not?" we asked.

Another procedure. More hospital time.

He left us, lasagne cooling. Terror gripping me. Matt reached over and took my hand,

"It is just a blood test and we will know."

"Know if I can go home and live, or stay here..."

Suddenly, I lost my appetite, and I curled up in bed and began to silently beg the universe to let them just be air bubbles and not subject me to more.

I just really want to go home.

That night, in the early dawn, I heard the nurse come in to take my blood sample. It was dark out, probably 5 a.m. This nurse was one of my favorites: young, gentle, and never asked questions. She quietly came in and took the sample by the reading light and was gone as quick as she came.

I laid in the dark, watching Matthew sleep in the cot beside me, and begged for mercy. *Please, let me go home. Please, let me escape this reality. This chaos.*

The next few hours were torturously long.

Dr. Hernandez's team was soon at the foot of my bed once more. Dr. Hernandez had a smile on his face as he announced that my white blood cell count was okay, and that he was able to release me. The date was Thursday, February 17th 2011, the day before my birthday. I grinned ear to ear and did not hear a word after that. Matthew was furiously taking notes down as his team rambled off all of the restrictions and rules that I would have to follow. No outside visitors. Any fever whatsoever and I would need to present to the emergency department and tell them to notify the General Surgery team. The list went on and on. I would need someone to remove my staples, return in two weeks for another CT, another appointment in a month, and close monitoring throughout. Mentally, all of this did not matter. I was going home and that is all that mattered.

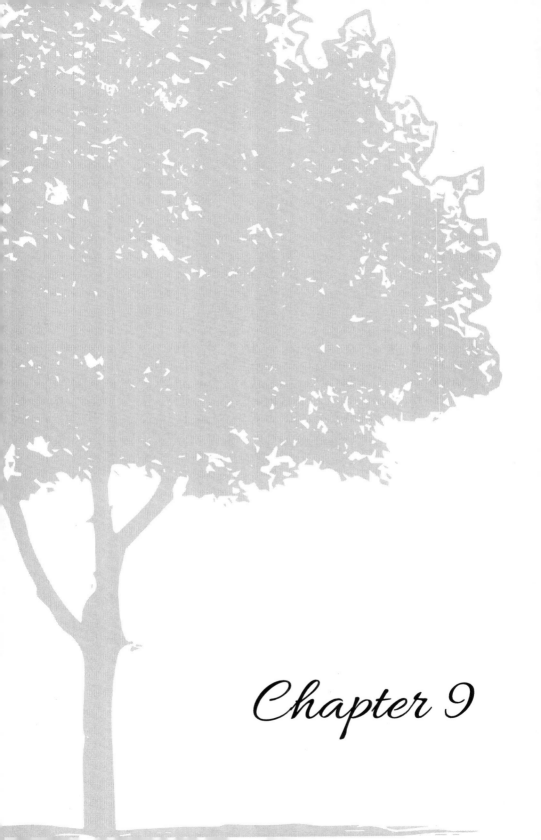

Chapter 9

Home

Matthew pulled into our driveway. The van lurched over the snow bank that built up after weeks of the snow plow coming by with no one coming to clean it away.

Putting it in park, the silence fell around us. Matt, wordless, gets out of the car and comes around to open my door. I take his arm and step out into the snow. He walks me gently around to the side door of the house. I step onto the back hall landing and I am frozen. My boots melting on the floor, I stand looking at the kitchen—the very same kitchen that was just filled with my family and friends.

It is empty. A serving bowl is still on the counter. Kim washed it and set it there. When Ava still lived.

"Do you need a hand?" Matt's quiet voice comes from behind me.

"No. Thanks." I slip off my boots and shrug off my coat. Stepping through the kitchen, I find my way to the living room sofa and sit.

Matt is doing runs back and forth to the van for all the flowers and our suitcases. So many flowers—over 30 bouquets in all—so many, that he needed a luggage cart to help him load them from our room down to the car.

I sat on the edge of my seat and stared into the blankness. The house was cold. Heat setting on low because we had been gone. I raise my eyes to meet Matt's and his say the same as mine.

This is not how it should be.

Hot tears burn my eyes. I look up and the shower flower arrangement is on the table. The house smells like catering. The house is as frozen as we are.

Matt closes the door and takes off his coat.

"Christ, it is freezing in here," he mutters. He goes over to the thermostat and begins punching in buttons. I sit, frozen as the air around me. There is no car seat. No little person to care for. Silence rings through the air between us. Matthew dutifully gets to work unpacking suitcases. He has never unpacked as soon as we came home from anywhere, but he is just as frozen as I am and desperate to do anything other than what we are.

I do not even know what this is.

I thought I would be more upset coming home. I thought I would howl and scream. Coming home was a scary thing, but this does not seem scary. This seems like home. Sitting on the edge of the sofa, I stare out the window. The snow falling just as it did when she was alive.

The world is continuing. Yet I am frozen.

"Cup of tea?" His soft voice interrupts my thoughts.

"Sure. Thanks, babe."

"Do you want to..."

I complete his thought in my head. Go downstairs. Yes. Very much so.

"Yes. Please. I want to sit by the fire."

"We should build a fort down there," Matt mutters.

"With a gun turret," I reply.

"And a moat. With alligators."

We share a quiet look and gentle smile. I just want to block out the world a while. I want to curl up and put my head on his chest. To find that little nook right underneath his collar bone, and put my head down in it until I can breathe once more. I want to turn off the phone, never turn on the Internet ever again. Maybe if I hide from the pain a while, it will help. Maybe.

I stand at the top of the stairs and look down them. They are steep. They have always been steep, old stairs. But now, so frail, I cannot put into words how I am supposed to do them.

"We could just stay upstairs." Matt's soft voice is behind me.

"No. The good couches are down there. And the TV and fireplace. Plus, there are no goddamned flowers."

He snorts. "Okay then. Let me set down the tea and come back for you."

He heads down the stairs solo, Charlie in tow behind him. Anger rises, and my face flushes with fury. I can't even go down the stairs alone? I stare down at my miserable body. First you kill my baby, and now you can't even waddle downstairs? Furious and fed up, I place my hand on the railing and grip it firmly. I place one foot on the stair below and slowly lower my weight. Looking down the stairs, my head spins. I grip harder and breathe through my mouth.

"No, dammit. I am doing this."

I see Matthew at the bottom of the stairs, frozen. He is scared, but sees my anger and determination. He says nothing as I slowly, meticulously waddle my way down the stairs. My staples pull, my ribs ache, and I am filled with body loathing at the weakness of it all.

I get to the bottom of the stairs and look around. The loveseat where I sat with my brother and sister, holding baby Leo. How I soaked that moment in and, like dust, it slips through my fingers. The gift table is still up in the corner. The gifts gone down. The room is cold and sterile, a stark contrast from the warm and safe embrace we built for her. Matt takes my arm and walks me over to the sofa; I look behind it and the playpen is gone.

"The playpen..."

"I took it down."

"By yourself?" In the reality of that moment, I look at his face and my eyes well with tears.

"Yah, it was awful. That damned mobile..."

Silence rings between us as I settle onto the sofa. No car seat, no baby to nurse. A body in ruins, and back to our new frozen reality.

We put on the TV and settle in.

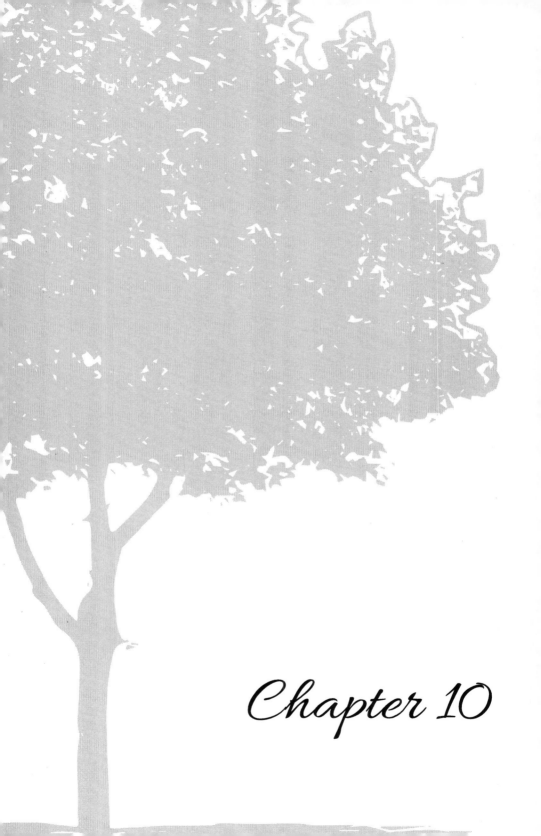

Chapter 10

Where Do I Belong?

Feb 22nd 2011

Dear Journal,

Today was supposed to be my first day of Mat leave. I am supposed to be sleeping in, folding baby clothes, and taking care of myself. Instead, I am planning Ava's funeral and recovering from a huge body trauma.

Part of me is so incredibly thankful to be alive. Just so grateful. I think of how close we came to Matthew being a widower and it makes me sick. I fought for him. I never want to leave him. Other parts of me are just so angry that everyone else gets to bring home their babies and I don't get to bring home mine. Why did my body do this?

The loss of potential and the idea of what our life would be is deafening. The door is there, shut with all of the baby things behind it, and it might as well have a big red flashing *light on the top. What do you do with the stuff? Especially when there is a very real chance it will never be used now ... I just can't see Matthew ever allowing there to be another baby... Hell, part of me is terrified.*

It's astounding how many people experience a stillbirth once you start to talk around about it. We really aren't alone, though it feels like we are the only people on the planet dealing with all this right now. Little comfort, but some comfort despite it all.

I love you Ava. I miss you, my darling girl.

I am weak, but growing stronger. As the days pass, I find the anger in my belly building. Angry that I am stuck in this body. Angry that I can barely climb the stairs without taking a breath. Angry that this is my life.

I hate my scars and everything they stand for. The liver scar is thick, hockey stick-shaped, and a foot long. The staple holes they said would fade aren't, and I look like I have a railroad going across my stomach. The lower corner of them pulls. It sits just above my hip bone, and every time I get out of a chair, or turn wrong, they pull and scream in pain. I loathe my body and all it has done to me. The Caesarean scar is cruel. Painful and thick, it is a cruel reminder of what was.

I am completely sick of this skin. Of living in this skin and existing in it. So I hide. Hide in the basement and watch ridiculous movies. Preferably ones where someone falls down a flight of stairs and the laugh track tells to you that it is funny. Something grotesque and crass in its humor. Something distractingly flashy and difficult to ignore.

I am on germ watch. Dr. Hernandez wants me to stay out of the public eye until he has cleared me with yet another CT scan at the end of the month. More testing. Even thinking about going back into the hospital makes the bile rise in my body. Panic, fear, confusion. I am not ready to go back in there.

We met with a loss educator that Shawn recommended. Her name was Carol. We managed to attend three of Shawn's prenatal classes before she was born. Three beautiful classes filled with hope and joy, and a friendship was formed. Matthew reached out to Shawn and asked for her advice of who could help us, and she gave us Carol's name. Soft and receptive, she came out to the house in the first few days of us being home. Carol listened, pained along with us. We told our story of losing Ava, and she nodded and breathed deeply as we told her all we had been through.

"I just do not know where to go from here," I said. "I do not know who I am or what do to with myself. I am in ruins and nothing... helps."

"This is your new normal, now. Your life now, after loss. And you need to take time to adjust to that," she responded.

The thought rattled—and comforted—me. This is our new normal, our new life without our daughter. It struck me in its simplicity and made me nauseated all the same.

All I could think was, "but I do not want this normal."

The midwives are ever present. Nikki, the soft English-speaking midwife, comes on my birthday and removes my liver staples. She brings me two beautiful flowers, one for Ava and one for me. Laura visits me weekly. She brings me comfort. She sits on my sofa and lets me rant and rave about the ignorant things people say. About how hard this is, how I just want her back. *I want Ava back.* It is every thought in my head and the answer to each and every question.

"How are you?"

"I want Ava."

"Can I get you anything?"

"Yes. Ava."

Matthew is possibly my worst offender. He asks me upwards of 20 times a day how I am. He is worried. He wants me well. He wants me to be okay. I am not okay. And I am sick of lying to him.

"How are you?" he asked as I quietly type on my computer.

"Fine. No, wait. I am not fine. My health is fine. I am not fine..." I sigh.

"Okay," he replies, timidly. He does not know what to do with that answer.

"Okay. New rule. You can only ask how I am 2 times a day. If you want to 'check in' with me, just say hi."

"Just say hi?"

"Yes. Just say hi. I will know that is your way of wanting to check in with me. I know you need to know how I am, but I can't answer 'how are you' one more time or I am going to lose my fucking mind."

He smirked at me and walked away.

At least the "how are you's" are only coming from everyone else in my life now. So many "how are you's."

The flowers are slowly dying and it is relief. With each one I throw out, it feels like I am being unburdened. Yet it scares me that it means she is disappearing. Like any remnant of her is disappearing. Matthew's work sent us a large bouquet of white lilies in a gigantic white ceramic vase. It has a grotesquely large cross on it.

I do not get it. Did they think we were Christian? Did they think God would comfort me now?

It is so gaudy, it is comical. Matt roared with laughter when he got home from work and saw it. Thankfully, it is funny because if it wasn't funny, I would have to throw it through a window.

I do not have a plan. I don't know what I am going to be doing. I was going to be a Mom. I am a Mom... a Mom with no baby. A Mom with no child. Now that I am not caring for our Ava, I have no idea what I am doing. I am dropping in weight like crazy. I don't know the last time I was this thin. So yeah, Matt is talking about going to the states to get me more clothes. Sounds great, sounds fun. Every idea that people come up with sounds great, but nowhere near as fun as having my child with me.

I feel as if there's a hole in my heart I cannot heal. I feel as if my heart isn't beating, as if there is no air in my lungs some days. How is it possible in today's day and age we didn't save her? How is it possible? Will I ever be whole again? She was perfect, but my body killed her. Blood pressure apparently killed her even though I didn't have high blood pressure. So many questions, so few answers.

Mommy did everything she could, Ava. I went to the doctor. I tried to save you. I thought you were okay until you weren't. Mommy did everything she could. I am so sorry I couldn't save you. Mommy's sorry.

This is by far the worst thing to ever happen to our family. Thank God I have Matthew

I woke up on the morning of the Dr. Hernandez CT scan appointment filled with fear. My hands shaking and my body quaking under the truth that they may find something noteworthy on this exam. They may need to do another procedure on me. This may not be the end of HELLP. Matthew took the day off of work to be with me. I didn't have to ask him. We are in simpatico these days; what I need, he knows, and together, we are walking this path.

I have to show up two hours before my appointment to drink the fluid for the test. That means arriving at the hospital at 7 a.m. It wouldn't matter what hour I had to get there. I was not sleeping much anyways. My biggest fear remained walking into THAT hospital again. The words of my mother were ringing in my head from our conversation the day before.

"Prepare yourself to go in there. The smell will trigger you. The sounds will too. Take your time and breathe through your mouth to avoid smelling the cleaners. The smell could bring on the memories for you."

In reality, the fear of more chaos was greater than anything else. The fear of them finding something that would cause them to need to rush me into another emergency surgery. Another moment without Matthew's hand in mine. Another day of chaos, of dying inside and being unable to stop it.

The drive to the hospital was silent. My hands sweating, my heart racing. "I just need to do this. Do this and it is over," is all that ran through my head. Whatever "it" is.

Matthew parked in the parking garage and came around to open my door. The simplest movements hurt still; three weeks after surgery, even opening a car door was impossible. He gave me his arm and me walked in.

Riding on the elevator down to the main level entry of the hospital, we were riding with an elderly couple. Obviously ailing, she had her husband's arm and a strong, stoic look on her face. She looks so much stronger than me. I feel ruined, and yet for all she could have seen in her life, she is strong. I feel gripped with terror and weak. I am humbled and angry all in the same instance.

As we walk from the parking garage, we step into the bright sunshine. A small pathway leads to the main doors. I go to glance right.

"Do not look down there," Matt says sternly.

I look up at him quizzically.

"The ambulance bay is down there."

Right. The same ambulance bay I would have been brought to. The same one where I was begging her forgiveness for her being born early. The one where she was dead and my world was about to crash down. I grip his arm hard and feel him steady himself under my grasp. Matthew opens the door for me and I meekly walk through it.

The smell of hand sanitizer is instant. I open my mouth and begin to take gulping breaths. Do not smell it, I beg my brain. *Do not smell that.* I find myself focusing on my feet and allowing Matthew to lead me down a maze of hallways. My faith completely rested in him, focusing on my breath.

We check in for my CT scan with little fanfare. They hand me a gown top and tell me to change and place my belongings in the lockers provided. As I walk to the changing area, my hands shake and I feel my soul begin to quake.

The last time I put on a gown, my world descended into madness. Matthew had to help me dress because of the screaming pain. And then, it all fell down. *It all fell down.*

I gulp back breaths and try to steady myself. My hands shake uncontrollably, so badly I can barely get myself undressed. I manage to get into the gown and step out of the changing area. Matthew is right there, his hand extended, the sweet man, as he helps me into a chair.

A nurse approaches and hands me the familiar jug of fluid. Same routine, drink this, do not urinate. You have an hour and a half.

As we settle in with my drink, Matthew is orienting me in the space. He tells me he knows who will be our tech today and that the room I will be in is at the end of the hall. He says he will speak with them so he can be present for the entire thing. I nod. Hot tears are in my eyes and I am willing them not to fall. I breathe and sip, breathe, and sip.

After an eternity of time passes, I hear commotion behind the doors Matthew says the scan will take place in. The staff begins to come in and out. My anxiety rises. This is it.

"Melissa?" My name is called by a young man in scrubs. His eyes are gentle. Matthew stands up behind me.

"Oh hey, man! How are you?" He walks by me and shakes Matthew's hand. They small chat about work and catch up, all the while, I stand and shake, trying to hide my terror.

"... my wife... trauma... stillbirth... please, take extra care and be as quick as possible." Matthew's voice is low and soft.

The man in scrubs gets tears in his eyes and comes up to me and offers me his arm.

"Now we are going to do this quickly for you, okay?" His voice mirrors Matthew's. I feel condescended to, something which would normally upset me greatly, but here, it is welcomed. I need compassion. I need gentleness. I am so broken. I hang onto my sanity by a thread as he walks me into the CT room and asks if I can get on the table. I can and he gently guides me into place and explains the IV solution they are starting in my arm.

He leaves my side and I find myself lying on the table, attempting to control the shaking of my legs. They need me to lay as still as possible. My breath is shaky and I am filled with the sensation to either scream, cry, or vomit.

"Just breathe," I tell myself. "Just breathe."

They say they are beginning the scan and ask me to hold as still as possible. Hot tears escape my eyes and pour down my cheeks. I can't hear Matthew's voice. I do not know if he is in the booth with them, but I pray this is over soon.

"I just need to readjust you." The young man returns and has me change position. He sees my tears and mercifully does not acknowledge them. I fear if he does, I may bust open at the seams.

Several more moments and the test is complete. Once again, the kind nurse comes and gives me his arm. Matthew is waiting by the door and I am ever-relieved to be back with him. I hurriedly change my clothes.

"Please, take me home." My voice is quiet and small. Matt says nothing as he buckles me into the car. Now we await the worst. What the test will find, we have no idea. But now we wait for three long days.

Life is long. Days pass as fast as molasses. Each day is the same repetition. E-mails from friends and family wanting to "check in." My anxiety builds up day by day, leading up to that appointment.

And then the phone rang one afternoon, while I am home alone, puttering by myself.

"Hello?"

"Hello, is Melissa there?"

Adrenaline rushed through me. The taste of metal filled my mouth. What now?

"Uh. Yes. This is her."

"Hi, Melissa. This is Sarah calling from Dr. McMillan's office. He has an opening this Friday and I understand you would like to see him?"

Dr. McMillan. The man who delivered Ava. The man who stood in scrubs with Dr. Hernandez, one of the surgeons that saved my life. I would finally get to talk to an obstetrician about Ava!

"Yes! I will take any time he is available. Any at all." All I want is just one moment to look at the man that delivered my daughter. To talk to any obstetrician that actually knows HELLP, knows us, knows my body. If I can ever trust my body to not kill me, I have to talk to a surgeon that knows it.

"10 a.m. is fine?"

"Yes! Thank you very much."

I did not even check with Matthew and his work schedule. It was going to have to do. I need to see this man and talk to him. This needs to happen. Now I will see Dr. Hernandez on Thursday and

Dr. McMillan on Friday. I may be completely fried with emotions by the time we are through.

Thursday morning, I woke up gripped with fear. Not about going back to the hospital. I knew I could do that now, but rather the news. What did the CT scan show and what does it mean from here? Going into the hospital was easier the second time. I knew I would be returning to the 7th floor, where I was cared for. I knew it would be hard, but I remembered the smells from a few days before and was prepared to handle them as such.

Walking into Dr. Hernandez's waiting room, I was shocked to see so many people there. We were given a number at check-in and were told to wait our turn.

And so we waited.

In the hospital, the cellphone coverage was spotty, but I was able to get just enough signal strength to send a message to my mom.

"Half an hour late so far. Full waiting room."

"Okay. Keep me posted." I can hear anxiety in her reply, palpable and strong. It occurred to me then that she was afraid. She was afraid about the results of this test, too. We were all on edge. I took Matthew's hand, shivering in fear. We sat side by side until finally, 45 minutes after our appointment time, my number was called to go back.

We were placed in a smaller exam room, with a big bright window. After the nurse took our information, she stated that the doctor would be in shortly. Unable to sit any longer, I walked over to the window. It was snowing. March 2, 2011 and the snow was still falling.

"Unending winter," Matthew muttered.

"Funny. I do not remember feeling cold in the car," I replied. Come to think of it, I can't remember feeling the weather at all. The cold doesn't bite anymore, yet it is still a harsh Canadian winter. Pausing on this fact a while, I stare out quietly, when the door suddenly opens.

It is the resident. The same resident that sent me for the x-ray and headlong into terror that Monday morning after Matthew mentioned fluid in my lungs. That same resident with poor bedside manner and a large ego. I glance at Matthew and see his face turn to steel. He is readying for battle and I want to cry. Here we go, once more.

"How are you?"

Loaded question. Let us keep this to the physical.

"Okay. Getting stronger. My staples came out. Some incision pain when I twist or pull."

"Well, let's take a look at that incision." He motions to the exam table and I oblige. Lifting my shirt, I expose the large, snaking scar. On each side of the scar are staple dots all along. He glances at my incision and feels along it with a cold efficiency. He asks a few more questions and says that he is going to review the CT with Dr. Hernandez and be right back.

He leaves, and Matthew and I sit quietly.

"One last wait to seal our fate," I say with a smile.

"Quality haiku."

"Quality with a k."

We banter back and forth, watching the snow. My legs are falling asleep and getting restless. My phone is buzzing in my purse. My Mom.

"Made it past the resident. Waiting for the big guy," I text.

"Keep me posted."

It is now an hour and fifteen minutes past our appointment time. We are weary and our emotions are wrung. Matt keeps checking his watch. I ask him not to, but cannot help glancing at the time whenever I can as well.

What could be taking so long?

There is a knock at the door. Mr. Resident pops his head in the door.

"Were you given antibiotics upon discharge?"

"Yes. I completed the course last week. They were a strong dose."

"Okay, thanks." He closes the door once more.

I glance at Matthew.

"Why would he not know that?"

Matt raises a knowing eyebrow at me.

"Okay, any reason other than that? Is there still an infection? Dr. Hernandez said that if there was still an infection, we may have to..." My voice trailed off.

"Do not go there. We aren't there yet." Matt's voice is firm.

Too late. My body begins to quiver and my brain races. He must think there is still some infection. That means more procedures. More hospital time. Tears fill my eyes and Matthew sees them. He reaches out and takes my hand. We sit in stony, anxious silence.

For an hour.

"Have they forgotten we are in here?" I ask.

Just before Matthew can answer, the door opens and in walks Dr. Hernandez. His face is bright and cheery. Wearing a plaid shirt and jeans, he looked remarkably relaxed. His energy instantly cut through the anxiety and tension that Matthew and I had building for the hour sitting there.

"Melissa, is that you?" he asked with an easy smile. He shook my hand with ease and sat down across from me. I looked down at my legs and saw my knees clacking together from terror. I drew them together and took a deep breath, sure that he could see my heart pounding in my throat from where he sat.

"So, everything is good." The tone was unclear. Was that a question? A statement?

"Is it?" I replied. I glanced back nervously at Matthew.

"Yes. Yes! I am sorry it took us so long. We had an emergency. But we took a look at your scans and everything is fine."

My brain could not understand this. Fine. What does fine mean?

"So the air bubbles?" I questioned.

"The air bubbles are gone. Everything is healing well. No further testing, no treatment." He shook his head no and the words hit my soul like a tsunami of relief. "I can hardly believe that is you. You look... look very good." His expression is warm and compassionate. It is true. I know I look, aside from the scars, the best I have in years. I have lost 30 pounds, my jeans are tucked into my riding boots as I sit, looking put together and poised. I hear this a lot. I have worked towards this image of me for close to 7 years and was unable to attain it. Now I lose what matters and I gain what doesn't.

"Thank you. I am getting there. I would like to begin physiotherapy when I can so I can get stronger."

"From six weeks from the surgery date, you can begin physio. I would like to see you again in 2 months, just to follow up." His warm brown eyes cheerfully dance on mine. He is trying to reassure me that things are okay. I am unable to hear anything but the coursing of blood through my body. I want to run from his office quickly, before they realize that they are reading the wrong scans and need me to be operated on. Before more suffering, more nightmares rush over me.

He shakes Matthew's hand and leaves the room. I quickly pick up my coat and throw my scarf on. Walking quickly past Matthew, I lead us out of the examination room. If I could run, I would.

"Hey, you, wait." Matt's voice is half-chuckling.

"Get me outta here."

"Roger. But hey, good news?" I turn to see his blue eyes relieved.

"Yes. Good news. Let's not tempt fate. Get me out of here."

We make our way quietly to the car. I call my mom from the ground floor to let her know that the results are good. She breaks down in tears, sobbing on the other end. My stomach rolls. The trauma is unending. I know she is nearly as ruined as I am, and here I am, leaning on her. This is all so screwed up.

Matt walks me back to the car. My burst of energy waning, I take his arm. Relief begins to pour over me and all I want to do is run back to the safety and security of our home. We do not say much on the way home.

The next morning, I woke completely exhausted from the trials of the day before. Of course, it was good news, but the idea of going back into yet another hospital, and this time we would be returning to the hospital they told me she had died in. Knowing how hard the day before was with all of its smells and sensations, I knew this one would be just as difficult—if not more so.

But I had to know.

Matthew worked from home for the morning, his work accommodating yet another appointment without any issue. I did not know if there were problems behind the scenes that he hid from me or if it really was going smoothly. All I knew is I was very comforted to have him with me each and every step of the way.

Dr. McMillan worked out of the Catholic hospital; the one where we labored and found out she had died. The drive into the hospital felt different this time. A calm fierceness ran through my veins. All this HELLP syndrome business aside, this appointment was finally about me, about her, and about our family. I needed to look at this man in the face and know that she was real and that someone would see this for something other than the fact that I had recovered.

Because I did not feel recovered.

Staring ahead at the road as we drove, I realized that our hands were linked. This is our new normal. Intertwined, constantly. He is now the only thing on this earth I have faith in.

"You know, this waiting room is going to rip us apart," I commented. "Strollers, pregnant bellies. Steel yourself."

"Hm. Lucky, innocent people. Great." The edge to Matthew's voice was cutting. We had to steel ourselves for these things. Something as innocent as a waiting room can cut to the core now. Gripping each other's hand harder, our eyes fix forward, knowing that pain awaits us.

Arriving at the hospital, Matthew led the way. I had no recollection of anywhere we were going, or what he was talking about as being familiar. I could see the pulse in his neck as we walked that told me his anxiety was heightened while being there. Suddenly, I felt horrid for having him along. It was me that wanted to see this doctor so badly.

"Babe?" I asked quietly.

"I got this," he muttered in response, holding a door for me in the long, sterile corridors.

Walking into the waiting room, I found myself staring at my feet, not wanting to look up and see what I knew would be there. I heard Matt snicker quietly and I raised my eyes to see what he was looking at.

The waiting room was filled with elderly people. Elderly women and spouses. In fact, we were the youngest people by a longshot.

"Are we in the right room?" I asked Matt quietly.

"Yup. The guy is the head of gynecology, not obstetrics, remember?"

Oh. Right.

Instantly, I felt my guard be lowered and a spring go back into my step. Check in went smoothly, and although I was terrified of having my blood pressure checked, I managed to move through it, and we were quickly brought into the meeting room.

"Wonder how long we will be here today?" Matt's comment rang with dark sarcasm.

"Anything less than yesterday and I will be happy."

With that, the door opened and in walked a face I recalled very well: Dr. McMillan.

With a firm handshake, I could see his face did not disguise his surprise to have me sitting in his room. After pleasantries were exchanged, he settled into the desk chair in front of me. He ran his hands over his hair and said plainly,

"Well, I am not too sure what you are here for..."

I let the silence fill the room as I attempted to find the real reason.

"Because. You were the first person to hold my daughter."

I could see the emotion on his face: one of compassion and fierceness. In one sentence, I took him back to our darkest moment together, and he took a moment to take it in.

"I have not had a gynecological follow-up. I have not been seen by anyone other than my midwives. I still do not know what HELLP syndrome is AND you held her. I had to see you." Tears caught in the back of my throat and I saw him suddenly sit up straight.

"You haven't been followed-up with?"

"No. Well, there were a bunch of doctors that came through when I was on the ward, and all offered to see me, but no appointments were set up. No one had examined me. Is that normal?"

"You require a 6-week follow-up." His voice filled with authority. "I would be more than happy to follow up with you late next month and take care of you." I felt myself relax into my chair—finally, someone to help.

He began to talk about HELLP syndrome and what happened with Ava. I tried to follow along with everything he was saying, but it was so complicated and my brain was overwhelmed. I could not stop staring at his hands, knowing those hands held my daughter.

Knowing, as I had heard from the midwives, how difficult that day was for him and for all the staff.

My eyes welled with tears at the thought.

"... stabilizing your bleeding, I was able to save your uterus..."

"You almost lost it? Were you called in because they did not know I would need a hysterectomy?"

His eyes said yes.

Taking a deep breath, I sat back further in my chair.

"But being able to save it does leave options for you in the future. As I have explained to your husband before, when you were asleep, you can have more children. Your uterus is healthy."

Tears poured down my cheeks; I could not believe what I was hearing. Matthew had said that Dr. McMillan had told him the very same before, but I did not believe it. Hearing those words, there is hope. I was overwhelmed.

"It is important you take this time. You need to heal. Emotionally, physically. Take a year. Get strong again, and then you can meet with the high-risk team and discuss it. If they are not able to take you, let me know and I will help you. I could help you. I have worked with families before and they have said the first 6 months, it is not wise to make big decisions. You need to grieve and heal. Take your time. And if you decide you want to do something more, let me know. I will help."

For the first time in a long while, I glanced up from his hands and saw his blue eyes and how genuine he was.

A year. A whole year? A whole year of this hell? My brain was overloaded and fraught with questions and concerns. I do not want to die. How could I contemplate another pregnancy, yet how can I not?

The meeting ends with booking a follow-up appointment in a few weeks time. All I can hear ringing through my head is "take a year… take a year…" on a repeat playback, over and over again. On the drive home, Matthew asks me what I am thinking and I simply do not know.

I am terrified of contemplating where we go from here, but to have a final timeline fixed to it may be even worse.

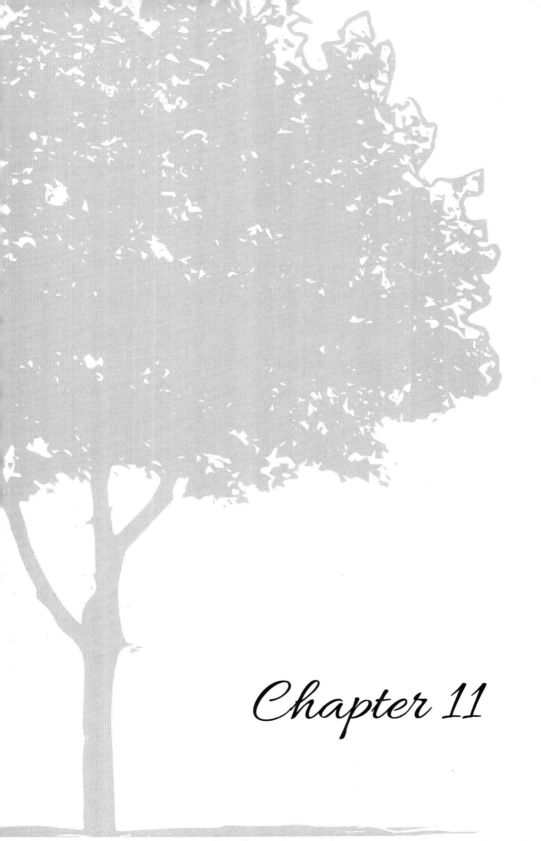

Chapter 11

Facing Fear and Living Without

Dear Ava,

I am watching that dog of yours go in circles, attempting to find a comfy place to lie down: circle, circle, circle, switch, circle, grumble, circle, grumble... flop. Ridiculous!

I continue to miss you each and every moment of each day. I find myself getting so mad at everyone and everything. I get mad when people do not realize how good they have it. Your Tante Kathleen, for example, who decided to be nitpicky over the type of dessert she wanted at Leo's baptism. Meanwhile, as I am listening to her tirade, all I can think is, I will never get to make you dessert. I never got to breastfeed you. I never got to play airplane or tell you to sit down at the dinner table. I never got to teach you to cook, or know what your favorite dish for your birthday would be. Other people get those things and I do not. Why don't I get to be happy like everyone else?

I get mad when people impose themselves on me. Impose their questions, their demands, their concerns on me. So many questions. I have been pelted with questions day in, day out. I can't take it anymore. Your Dad has taken to simply rephrasing to limit the questions for me. He has been asking me each and every day how I am, not realizing the pressure it is putting on me. He now simply says "Hi, person," as a way of letting me know he is worried.

Five weeks since we lost you. Five of the most horrible weeks of my life. I still count my life in weeks, soon to be months, and then years of missing you. I fear with each passing week, people will forget or continue to wish that we would move on. I do not wish to move on. I mourn you. I miss you. I want my baby Ava back so bad I can barely function.

The ache I feel for you is impossibly painful. As if a deep cavern has been carved into my soul, I feel as if I am standing on the edge of this cavern, knowing madness lines the bottom, and debating whether to jump. To descend down the rabbit hole of missing you or fight to stay here and sane. I am beginning to lose my will to fight, beginning to shut down, begin to numb and give in. I have the right to be the crazy lady whom never recovered from losing you. It's my right, my cross to bear.

I won't, though. I hang on for you. I want your legacy to be one of healing. I do not want your story to be that Mommy and Daddy fell apart and were never okay again. I do not want your story to be one of pain, insufferable agony that engraves scars onto the soul. I want you to know that we loved you enough to hang on to you. We loved you enough to risk my life to have you. We loved you so much that we live each day for you, so you can see the world through us, so we can take you with us to every single place we go.

Mommy misses you, darling girl. I miss you so very, very much. I ache for my daughter. The darkest, deepest pain possible.

I love you, Ava. I have loved you since the first time I told you walking around the grocery store. I will always love you and miss you, darling girl. You will always be in my heart.

Love,
Mama

The door to her room is closed. All day, Matthew is gone to work and it remains closed. I walk by it for what feels like hundreds of times a day. The most treasured possessions of my life exist behind that door, and yet, I cannot bear to open it. I feel like my innocence is locked in there, along with the fresh smell of happiness.

I do not remember what joy feels like.

Most of my days feel numb. I am lost. I am without purpose or direction. I do not have a job. I do not have a baby. I am a childless mother and there is no sense in this. I cannot wrap my head around where I belong, but I know, without a doubt, that I do not belong anywhere.

The door is taunting me. I know, at some point, I need to open it. I know it cannot remain closed forever. Our house is too small, so we need every inch we have. I have had offers from family and friends to help me. My mom has offered to clean it out, but I know this is my job. I know I must do this for her.

But I am just not ready to. Her due date was approaching quickly. I felt a rumbling beneath my feet, but I simply cannot fathom this year. Her due date was a Tuesday. Every woman knows the two dates of her pregnancy that she repeats the most; the first day of her last period and her due date.

The beginning of March was cruel. All those conversations I had came flooding back to haunt me. Each person's guess: "Oh, I think the baby will come on the 6th," "This little one will be early," and "Oh, it is your first. This baby will be here the end of March." And with each date that passed, and she wasn't being born, my heart broke a little bit more. As if that were even possible. I never thought about dates like this before. Dates were now all-consuming. March 8th 2011 was one month after she had died.

I woke up that morning in a daze. I ran my hands over my still belly and breathed.

"One month. Happy birthday, Ava." I curled onto my side and sobbed. It was a miserable day. My parents surprised me by coming for lunch, and I walked through it, broken. Each smile, forced. Each movement, weighted down. My arms ached and felt like lead. The entire time, I willed myself to remain present while wanting to curl up in bed and cease to exist.

I know they did not realize the date. Dates matter now. Each day is another without her and is another reminder that I do not have her here. I am stalked by "should be's." My life remains a figment of what it should be.

But it will never be again.

Her due date came quietly in the night. There was nothing remarkable about that day. We ate the same frozen meal that we had been eating for weeks, which were care packages dropped off by anyone and everyone. My phone did not ring, wondering if I had the baby yet. Nothing was as it should have been. I continued to ignore her room and wonder just where I belonged now.

My ribs ache every day. I feel the need to support them when getting up and moving around. I need to just be patient and "heal." Whatever the hell that means.

Our first session with our counselor, Kathy, was a month after Ava passed away. Matthew and I had attended Kathy for sessions before in the past, before we were married, for pre-marital counseling and the like. We trusted her and knew she would know how on earth to put us back together again. Matthew did not protest going whatsoever. Both of us knew we needed to. In the hospital, I had turned to him and said that we were going to need to see Kathy, and I was right.

It was a month after coming home from the hospital; I was walking into our bedroom. Suddenly, I flashed back to the morning of her shower. Getting out of bed, feeling horrific, holding my side, and wondering why I was so sore.

Regret.

Guilt.

I broke out in a cold sweat and my heart began to race. I sat myself down hard on the floor and gripped my chest. I must be having a panic attack, is all I could think. But was I?

I buried my nose into my knees and willed myself to breathe slowly. Slowly and surely, the room stopped spinning and just as it did, I began to cry.

"I must be crazy," I said aloud through tears. Simon the cat wandered over and rubbed on my foot. "I need help."

One week later, Matt and I were in Kathy's office, our hands linked between us, ready to face the demons together.

We dove right into EMDR therapy. EMDR is an effective trauma therapy that uses both sides of your brain simultaneously to unlock and recode how your brain processes events. It was fast, effective, and emotionally hard as hell.

First and foremost, Kathy led me through the most horrifying moments, of finding out she had died and of the hospital, the mere thought of which could lead me into a frenzy of emotions and panic. It would take months of intensive work to break the cycle of chaos in my mind, but slowly, I was set free of it, and the grief was allowed to follow behind it.

"I just want to go up to the roof and scream." Matt's voice is harsh and dark. We are in the midst of a session of therapy with Kathy. Kathy leans back in her chair, her fierce bright eyes fixed on Matthew. Matthew is talking about the chaos of the hospital on the night Ava died, when all hope seemed lost and my condition was ever deteriorating.

"Then do so. Your mind does not know where you are. Go there in your mind, to that room, and imagine yourself doing just that. Walk up to the rooftop and scream."

The look on Matthew's face is one of disbelief. I see him settle into the idea and he pauses, and with the guidance of eye movements from Kathy's guidance, he begins to process. I sit beside him and watch, captivated. I see his jawline is strong and angry. Suddenly, his shoulders drop slowly, his eyes well and I feel a tension released.

Kathy glances at me and then back at Matthew. All I can think of is relief for him and ever-present knowing that we are going to be so screwed up for so long.

One sunny morning, I woke up and the sun was streaming in our bedroom windows. I reached over to Matthew's side of the bed and found it empty. Another work day and he is gone out to work. The days meld together for me. I can only tell the days of the week from when he is in bed when I wake and when he isn't. I blink into the brightness and follow the line of sunshine. It streams across the bed and into the hall. The hardwood floors gleam as the sunbeam comes to an end at her bedroom door, across the hall from our room.

I get out of bed, careful to support my ribs as I stand. I shuffle-step to her door, place my hand on the knob and open it.

Instantly, the smell of fresh paint hits me. Fresh paint and cardboard boxes and the glue from her crib. The smell assaults my nostrils as I stand, staring into her room. The room said it all.

The mental image of Matthew returning to the house alone. The house, filled with shower presents, and the pack-and-play lovingly set up. The house where we just celebrated her. As he probably stood there with the snow dripping off his boots, his wife in a coma, he was affronted with the contents of this room. And he took it all down himself. He put it all away.

He packed up the playpen, as it played its lullaby tune.

He packed up the car seat, boxes, onesies, and stuffed them into this room. And he shut the door.

Standing there, it was apparent what that moment was. Hurried and pained, I could barely open the door fully for not hitting the contents in the tiny bedroom. The pile was high in front of me to the crib.

I stood and stared a while, and with great sadness, I closed the door.

The dream of my life is in that room.

Later that morning, I walked by the room again and opened the door. I stood and stared for the longest while. I sank down on the hardwood floors and stared. Simon came by and curled up beside my legs. Suddenly, without warning, I felt gumption rise up in my belly and found myself striding into the room. Pulling out the car seat box first, I began to sort things through. Not wanting to identify with the items individually, I blindly sorted through them. All clothing would be kept and stored. I refused to make any final decisions on anything. I could not bear the thought of separating from any of her things, but some realistic changes had to be made. Clothing boxed, open diapers and wipes set aside for donation, and the larger items had to find some space in this room to exist so I could just be in there.

I just want to be in her room. I just want to be sitting in her chair. I just want to be doing what I should be doing, with her.

My pace picked up, moment by moment, furiously sorting, blindly identifying and moving through the moments of what was needing to be done. Over the course of an hour, I managed to box all the clothing, pack the closet filled with items, and begin donation boxes. Suddenly, I turned around and saw the ashes sitting in her crib. Her paperwork was in it.

My heart went still. The paperwork. What is that? Thinking back to the day we picked up her ashes, they handed Matt an envelope. What was that? Walking over tentatively, I picked up her ashes and held them close to my heart. Setting them down gently, I picked up the paperwork. Opening it tenderly, I begin to scan it.

Certificate of cremation.

Date of death: February 8th 2011

Date of cremation: February 18th 2011.

My birthday.

I gasp.

She was cremated on my birthday.

I gasp!

Oh, God!

The room spins and I clutch the crib to steady myself. It is too late. I am going down to the floor, hard. I fall to the floor in a blazing daze. The cremation certificate falls out from my grasp and I reel onto the cable fibre of the carpet.

A guttural, primal scream radiates from my soul. The wail of loss, the lost Mama, screaming in hell for her baby. They burned my baby on my birthday? On my damned birthday! Why!? Why would they wait 10 days!? Why, of all days, did it have to be my birthday that they cremated her? All-consuming grief overcomes me and I am lost into disorienting, blinding torment of loss and agony.

Ding-dong!

What? Was that the door? I wipe my tears and realize my face has been pressed into the carpet of her room. How long have I been crying?

Ding-dong!

"Hey, Mouse?" a loud, friendly voice calls. It is my Dad.

Dad? Of all moments! Dad never drops by. I wipe my tears furiously. How, of all moments, is this the moment that he drops by?

I will myself off the floor, get up, and walk past the boxes and the chaos and into the kitchen. I glance at the clock on the way by. It is nearly lunch.

"Hey, Dad."

I round the corner into the kitchen and catch his eye. His face drops from a smile into instant concern, and I fall into his arms, sobbing.

He says nothing, and just stands and holds me. I manage to squeak out the words.

"Cremated. On. My. BIRTHDAY." I bury my head into his coat and I feel him brace himself against my torrent of tears.

"Ah, love." He knows that there are no words for this moment.

My tears slow and the moment begins to ease. I hear him talking about lunch and getting out into the sunshine a while. I nod and say I will go wash my face.

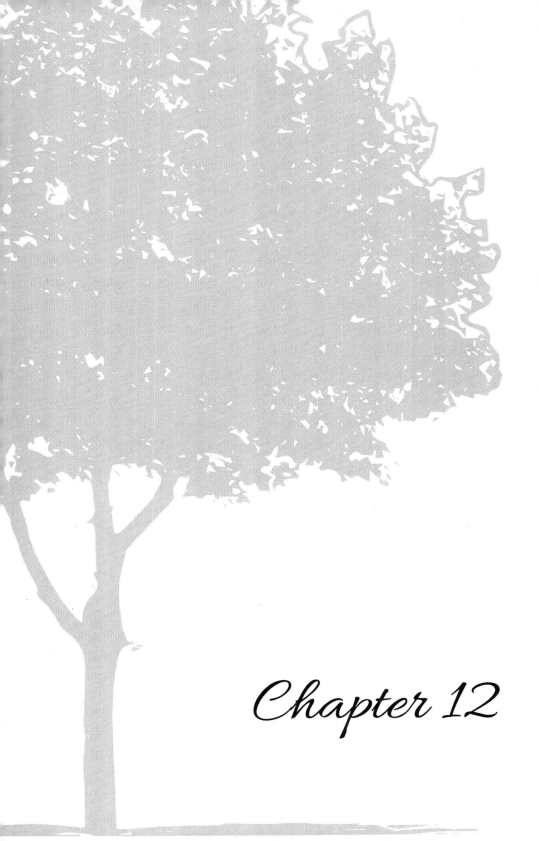

Chapter 12

Memorialized

Everyone keeps saying we should have a memorial.

I cannot even fathom that she is gone because it barely seems like she was here sometimes. It is like a dream. I dreamed I was going to have a baby, and then that dream turned into a nightmare.

It is just, I cannot figure out if I am asleep or awake.

Laura comes for a visit and asks if we have thought about making any "arrangements." Certain words have come into my life since Ava died. Arrangements are one of them. Is it like flowers? Because we have plenty of those. Weeks afterwards, I am still throwing out flower arrangements. And they are not ending, including the gigantic bouquet of white lilies with the large cross on the vase that Matthew's work sent one month after she died. Apparently, we are Christian or maybe just the vase is? I am not sure. All I know is God and I are not on speaking terms.

Maybe that is what makes this decision so hard about the "arrangements" we have to make. Most people turn to their place of worship and follow the program that is laid out for them. They seek counsel from the faith leader who married them, whom they have turned to in strife for their entire lives. We do not have that. Further, even if I did, what use would it be? I was on strict restrictions for the longest time to stay away from crowds, and the last thing I want right now is a crowd of people judging my grief.

When Laura asked, I knew the question was coming. It was the same question my mother had asked a few times, as well as my sister. The same question Matt and I muttered to each other in the dark at night,

"What should we do for her?"

"Nothing seems adequate."

And that says it all. Nothing is adequate. Nothing is enough to honor our lost daughter. How do you have a burial without a cemetery? There is little I know of what I desire to do for her, but I do know I do not want her in a cemetery. Instantly, my mind flashes back to the ICU bed. She is lying in Matthew's arms, and I reach over to touch her skin. She is ice cold. I cannot fathom another thing of hers being as cold as she was in that moment. I do not want to visit a cemetery and tend to it. I do not want that in my life.

"I do not know yet," is all I could respond to Laura. She did not press and our conversation moved on. Matthew and I exchanged a glance, and I knew we would further it later.

That night, Matthew came up from the basement with yet another frozen lasagne from the oven.

"And for tonight's delicacy, we have yet another dodgy lasagne!" He waved his arms in front of it like he was showcasing car.

"Oh! And let me guess; I will make a salad?" I said, fighting a smile.

"Yes! And we will push it all around our plates, barely eating, while watching another Will Ferrell movie."

"Sounds about right," I said. He side-glances at me as he sets to work and I take a breath.

"So, the arrangements..."

"Yes." He does not even look up from the stove.

"I am going to call Wayne."

"Yeah," Matt nods slowly. "That makes sense. Does he do these things?"

"I think so. I do not know. Either way, he will know what to do."

And he did. Coming into our home one evening that week, Wayne knew just what to say and do. He helped guide us with compassion and honest friendship. It was with his suggestion that we began to see that we had a choice to make in regards to Ava's life. He asked us:

"What do you want?"

The only response that made sense was life. I wanted her to live. I wanted her legacy and story not be that her family fell to pieces and never recovered. I wanted her to be remembered and celebrated. I wanted her life to be present in ours.

"If you want life, why not do something living? Like a tree."

It was an instant fit; a tree to be planted in her honour. Something living we can tend to, something tangible and alive.

After Wayne left, I decided to see where I could have a memorial tree planted. Being that I did not want a cemetery, my first inclination was to contact the local parks department. I was flatly told that memorial trees were "no longer done," and that I was welcome to join in a memorial wall they had at a local park.

"But then it will be just like a cemetery," I said to Matt, that night, with tears in my eyes.

"Maybe they just didn't understand. Maybe they had a bad day. People hear dead baby and they panic, and just want the conversation to end. Try again tomorrow," Matt advised.

I was still too angry to see his side of things. Why does it have to be so difficult? I just want to have a place for my daughter. It took about a week for me to build up the gumption to call again, and this time, I tried a different tactic. Having worked with the city in the past, I decided to pull that connection and make the call as a "former employee" of the city.

"Hi! Kristen? This is Melissa Krawecki. I used to work down at the works department. How are you?"

"Oh, I am fine. How are you?"

"Well, it has been very hard. I am not working for the city right now because my daughter died."

"Your daughter died?"

This is the exact same person I just spoke with a week earlier. You think you would remember someone's child dying. I swallowed hard and continued.

"Yes, she was stillborn. My family would like to have a memorial tree planted in her honor. Nothing showy. It does not have to have a plaque or anything. I was thinking just a tree my family can plant together and visit from time to time when they need. What are your thoughts?"

"Well, we do not really do memorial trees anymore..."

I let the silence hang.

"... But we are doing a bunch of new plantings at Waterworks Park. I am sure we can make that possible to you."

My heart leapt. She gave me the information. She would be able to allow me to pick the species of tree we wanted, provided it was native to the area. In addition, she would allow us to pick the location of the tree under her guidance and knowledge of the area. Being that it was already March, and planting season was beginning soon, she thought it best we be able to come up with an answer quickly for her.

I thanked her profusely and promised to contact her back. It was the first glimmer of hope that I had felt in a very long time. Maybe, just maybe, we would be able to have something fitting for our girl.

When Matthew came home from work that night, I was triumphant. I had gone online and printed out gigantic lists of all the native tree species along with pictures. We sat down at the dining table and poured over them for nearly an hour.

"This tree is a tulip tree. It has big beautiful flowers. Quite girly but its blooms are fragile and it is a bit messy," I said, reciting what I had read for hours that afternoon.

"I think the tree should be a bit girly." Matt's voice was soft. "I mean, it is for a girl."

"So is the dogwood out on the name alone then?"

"Here is our daughter's dogwood? Yes, that is out," Matt snickered. "Any other choices there?"

"Well, there is the sunburst locust, which is bright yellow in the spring. Very joyful looking and it darkens over the summer. No flowers though. I think I want flowers."

"Yup," Matt agreed.

"There is the Eastern Redbud. Mom and Dad have one in their backyard. Look at this picture of it. It gets lacy, purple flowers that line the trunk. Very delicate flowers. And it looks like the entire tree glows in flowers. And their leaves are heart-shaped."

"Heart-shaped flowers?" Matt asked.

"Yeah. See?" I held up the picture print out for him to see.

"I like this one."

"Me too."

We woke up on the morning of her service filled with nerves. We met with our immediate family on a warm May morning. The sun shone bright and the park was quiet. There was a peace that filled the air, along with a reverence for the importance of this moment. This was Ava's moment and no one else's. Our commitment to having this be a moment focused on her, and thus, our desire for only a few in attendance, was immediately affirmed when we looked out and saw the genuine love in each person's eye.

With Wayne's guidance, we planted and watered her tree. Each person brought a special something for her. It was filled with love and quiet adoration of her, as we gently said goodbye to our girl.

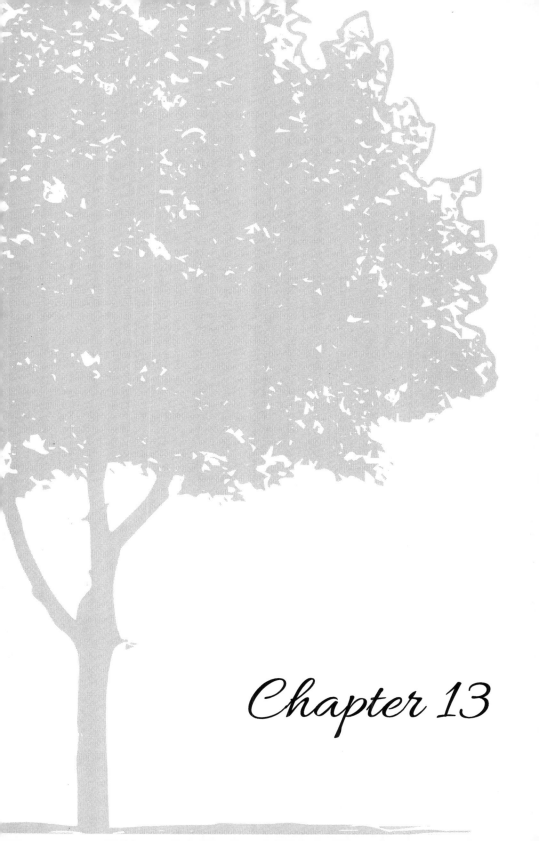

Chapter 13

Return to Life

"Work called today."

"They did?" Matt looked up from his computer as I stood in front of him.

"Yeah. They said that they have an opening and were curious if I would be ready to come back to work."

"Hmm." Matt said nothing, his expression blank as his eyes met mine.

"I think I am ready to go back to work. After all, I kind of lost everything here."

"Ava, your job, your identity..." His voice trailed off.

"Yeah. All of it. I lost all of it. I am worried that I am not strong enough to work. Like, what if I break down crying? What if people ask too much..."

"But your work has been very supportive. Very, very supportive. That is a plus." Matt has a gift of walking both sides of an argument equally, without showing signs of preference. Not until I ask him directly, will I know what his opinion is.

"What do you think I should do, Matt?"

"I want you to do whatever you want to do. If you want to stay home, you can stay home forever. I never care if you work another day in your life, truly. I just want you to be happy. Well, as happy as we could ever be anymore. If working makes you happy, then work. If staying home makes you happy, then stay home."

"So, you are claiming neutral territory on this one?"

"No. I am on your side."

"I need to do something. I think work might be good."

And that was it. I returned to work two weeks later. Back to my old office and the compassionate embrace of my coworkers. It was not always easy. In fact, there were some days where I was nearly torn to shreds by innocent, well-intentioned banter. The first two weeks nearly undid me at the seams. I sobbed to and from work each and every day, and would need to walk the block on my breaks just to regain my composure. Having to keep face that I was okay when I was not was exhausting, but it needed to be.

Slowly coming back into life, we were a shell of our former selves. This new normal felt like a life sentence we were given, punished and sanctioned for the rest of our lives. Both of us found ourselves increasingly restless, wanton, and driven into life. We wanted to live. Wanted this to have some sort of outcome or purpose.

"I can see why people sit on talk shows and say 'it all happened for a reason,'" Matt said to me one morning,

"Because pain needs purpose?"

"Yes. Purpose and reason."

"Have you found purpose yet?"

"Nope. You?"

"There will never be a good-enough reason."

It was our truth. There will never be a good-enough reason. After seeking the recommendations of Dr. Hernandez and Dr. McMillan, who assured us a second pregnancy was possible, we thought it prudent to investigate the issue more thoroughly. Matt said he had met the head of obstetrics when I was in hospital, and Laura worked with him as an employee. She recommended that we meet with him to discuss our options as he worked with high-risk patients.

It took months to get the appointment. Months of calling his office for no response. Frustrated and exasperated, I contacted the midwives' office and asked for their assistance in making the referral.

I had an appointment at the end of the week.

Burned, bereaved, and beyond recognition of our former selves, we walked into the appointment hopeless and wondering why we were putting ourselves through this ordeal. In no condition to consider a subsequent pregnancy, I needed to know from the highest authority possible that the option was still on the table, so to speak.

I wrote down a list of questions for him, my notepad dutifully on my lap.

"Do you think he will recognize us?" I asked Matt.

"Not a chance. It was half a year ago and you look nothing the same anymore. And me, I am forgettable."

Well, half that sentence was true. I did look completely different than before at half my former size.

"You are far from forgettable," I murmured.

Dr. Natale walked into the room and I immediately recognized him. Short stature, grey-haired, with scrubs on and a white doctor's coat. He came in and shook our hands, in a business-like fashion, and set my chart down on the desk in front of him.

"I understand you have been wanting an appointment. What can I help you with?" His manner was cool and professional.

Is this guy kidding himself? What can he help us with? I instantly wonder if he is really the all-knowing, amazing, high-risk doctor everyone told me about.

"Well, um," I struggled to contain the tremble in my voice. "I am Melissa and this is my husband, Matthew. I had HELLP syndrome in February this year. We had Dr. Dewitt. My daughter Ava died. I almost died." Tears bite the back of my throat. "And everyone said I should talk to you because you are the most skilled obstetrician in cases like mine."

Suddenly, the facade of his face falls. I see shock and palpable sadness flush across him. He leans forward heavily, mere inches from me.

"YOU are Melissa? You?" He shakes his head bewildered and stares at Matthew. Rising to his feet, he puts out his hand and earnestly takes mine and shakes it softly this time. "Melissa. Of course. Of course, I remember you. I am so very sorry." He takes Matthew's hand and says the same to him. "I am very sorry for your loss, Matthew."

"Thank you."

"We need to know if it is possible. We need to know if we are mourning the loss of being parents at all along with her." I look at him, raw and open.

He takes a deep breath and begins to look through the file before him. Logging onto the computer, he goes through my electronic records.

"Have you ever been tested for blood clotting issues?"

"No."

He goes through and takes a complete medical history, as well as reads all the records for Dr. Hernandez, Dr. McMillan, and Dr. Dewitt.

"We will need to run testing of your blood to see if you have any blood clotting disorders and I need to visualize your liver with an ultrasound to ensure its health. Having more children is always an option. Percentages with no blood clotting disorders are around 10-15% chance of a reoccurrence of HELLP, 25% chance of preeclampsia on setting. That is if you are healthy. We will need to heavily monitor the pregnancy. You will have to listen to me. Do as I say. Be prepared to stay with us in hospital, and be prepared to face the triggers of it all. It is possible. I can assist you with that."

"What would the pregnancy look like?" I asked.

"We will need to know the results from your blood labs. However, we would be watching your placenta closely. We do not know what causes preeclampsia. However, we do know that the placenta is a factor. We would want to increase the blood flow and monitor the blood flow closely between yourself and the placenta. We would do an ultrasound early in the pregnancy, as well a dating ultrasound would be prudent, in case we have to take the baby early, so we know exactly how far along you are. In wanting to increase the blood flow, we have seen great results in having you take a blood thinner and low-dose aspirin, starting at 10 weeks. We would stop the blood thinner before the birth, at approximately 36 weeks. HELLP syndrome onsets after its first presentation. Therefore, at around 34 weeks, we will monitor your blood pressure and condition closely. If HELLP syndrome is coming, I will know it."

Taking a deep breath, he sat back from his computer and looked at us closely.

"This is a leap of faith. You have to want it and I am going to need you to trust me. You are going to have to do as I say and keep yourself as calm as possible. Having a pregnancy after loss is very, very difficult. You need to trust me and abide me. If it is in your heart to have another child, I can help you."

His authority and calmness were captivating. It was all so much to take in. I knew any pregnancy would have to be considered one day at a time. It was all too much to wrap my mind around. Matthew was furiously taking notes, which is good, as I doubt I could remember much more than the tone of his voice and the feeling in this room.

We thanked him for his time and he gathered up my file. Before he turned to leave, he came over to me again and, once more, shook my hand.

"Please, let me know what you decide to do. I remember Ava. I was able to see her when you were in hospital. She was stunning. Very beautiful. You were so sick, so I can't make any promises, but I can assure you, I will take very good care of you."

And with that, he was gone.

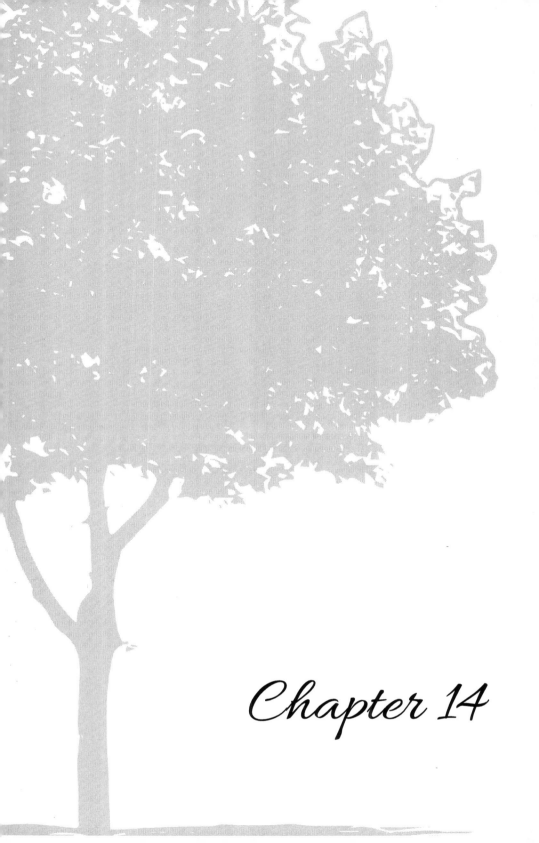

Chapter 14

Leap!

We made the decision to have another child in the middle of the pouring rain on Manhattan Island in New York City.

We had gone there to get away over her 6-month birthday. We had gone to clear our head, to breathe, to love, and to come to the decision we never thought possible. From the moment we walked out of Dr. McMillan's office, we took his advice very seriously: one year. We took 6-months to collect ourselves, for me to get stronger, and for us to lean against each other and each, as individuals, come to know what we had to do.

I saw the decision before me as impossible. It was as if we were standing on the top floor of a burning building. The smoke was rising and we knew we could not linger. We had to make the decision of either leaping from the building, a decision that could cost us our lives and yet save us all at the same time (having another baby), or we could walk back down through the smoke and the flames together (not having another baby.) Either way, we would hurt. Either life would demand great courage.

I grappled with the decision quietly within myself. I never discussed it at therapy or even spoke of it to anyone at length. Slowly, as time went by, as days turned into weeks, and as we slowly and painfully approached the 6-month mark, a slow seething anger grew in my belly.

I hated my life.

I hated getting up in the morning and not having her to care for.

I hated the fact that we were "free" to do as we wished.

I hated our new normal in each and every way.

There was not a single day where I reached its end and felt contentment. I was furious that this was my new life and saw our life with no children as a spirally bottomless hole.

I knew, deep down, that if I did not try, if I did not leap, that I would die spiralling.

But to ask Matthew for his support to put my life on the line? To ask Matthew to be my rock as we leap together? To begin to put together the plan of how we would even go about having another pregnancy was simply unfathomable. I needed him to make the decision for his heart alone. This was not something I wanted to coerce him into. This was not something I even wanted to debate. I knew what I needed to do, but I could not even comprehend the conversation if we did not agree.

It was in New York City that I knew we would find out each other's decision. I knew what my answer was, and I was afraid to say it out loud.

On our second night in NYC, we had decided to go for dinner early and enjoy walking around out of the hot sun. It was a long August day, very hot and humid. As the sun went down, the harshness of the day began to subside, dark clouds overhead giving a welcome reprieve from the day's heat. We walked out of the restaurant, hand in hand.

"I think it is going to rain," Matt said. I could smell the rain too. "Maybe we should take a shortcut back? I didn't bring the umbrella."

"Ah, I am not made of sugar. I won't melt." I smiled up at him, like I could care about a little warm August rain.

We managed to get around five blocks when, suddenly, the skies opened up and it began to pour.

"There's a store there," Matt pointed. "We could go and shop and get out of the rain."

"Sure," I replied loudly over the sound of the rain. Just then, the light turned and we had to wait for our opportunity to cross. Matt stood behind me, attempting to shelter me from the rain. I leaned back into him and suddenly, I heard him say,

"I need to try again. I need to have another baby." His voice was small and soft and incredibly sad.

I turned around and saw his face staring at his shoes. I lowered my face to meet his and replied,

"Me too."

We took each other's hand and did not say another word on the long and wet walk back to the hotel.

We spent the rest of the trip sightseeing and ruminating on what the plan would be. How would we pull this off, assuming we could get pregnant again? We had already seen the worst and were well aware that it could all go wrong.

Dr. Natale was our obvious choice to drive any future pregnancy. I felt safe with him. He was the Chief, so I felt as though he would be respected by those also assigned to my care. Additionally, his authoritative nature was appealing. I wanted to be able to learn to trust a doctor again, and I felt as if he had the greatest chance of enabling me to do that. Dr. Natale had also assured me that he could keep Dr. McMillan and Dr. Lopez apprised, bringing together a knowledgeable team and support system for me. I would also need Laura. There was just no way around it. I was going to need her. I could not imagine doing this again without her. I felt I needed her to act as a liaison between the hospital and me. To help me understand and to aid me when I felt trauma setting in. I needed her protection, advocacy, and mostly, I needed her to see this next chapter in the journey with me.

"Are you going to have another baby?" was possibly the most frequent question I was asked. Right after, "Oh, what happened?" I knew that having to tell the story, explain what was going on and why, would cause me significant stress. That meant we had to tell as few people as possible about the baby, and to simply say what I need, whenever I needed it. If that meant not telling each and every ultrasound technologist "the story," then I needed Dr. Natale to communicate that.

Most of all, to keep it low key. Keep our focus on one thing and one thing alone; healthy Mama and baby. No fuss. No drama. Just us.

Five months later, as the ball dropped on 2011, we felt we had a plan in place. We felt we had given ourselves a year with our Ava. We felt as ready as we were ever going to be to take the leap into a new life.

I found out I was pregnant on a Friday. We had flown home from Quebec City the day before. That week was Ava's 1st birthday, and deep down, I knew that I was pregnant. But I couldn't dare take a test around her birthday. It was Ava's year, Ava's day with her Mom and Dad, and I couldn't confuse my grief with the gigantic onslaught of emotion that would be thrown at me upon finding out we were expecting again.

I woke up early that Friday morning with fear in my belly, and I padded my way to the bathroom. Matt was asleep, but I knew he would hear me getting up. I knew he would know what I was doing. I took the test, my hands shaking and I stared at lines. Not being able to bear the moment, I turned it over and placed in on the counter beside me. The last year flashed in front of my eyes, in perfect cinematic Hollywood-style playback. Waking up in the hospital, our tears and fears, her memorial service, Matt's smile, and kissing him in the middle of a rainstorm until we got to here. This baby would be part of all our story. I cautiously and ever-so slowly turned over the test.

Two pink lines.

I stared down at them and felt nothing.

"How can I feel nothing?" I asked myself. Staring, I thought of all that this next year would entail, and what road we are on now. My hands went to my belly and I stared up at the mirror, standing in the exact same spot I was when I found out I was pregnant with Ava.

"Oh. Here we go." Quietly, the words passed my lips.

I opened the door, test in hand, to find Matthew tying his robe in the hall right outside the bathroom door. His eyes met mine and they were ardent. Seeing him made me laugh instantly; the moment felt so huge, it was ridiculous, and I felt laughter rise from my belly.

"Well!" I laughed, handing him the test, "Here we go again!"

"Are you kidding me?"

"Nope."

I barely got the words out as his large, heavy arms draped across my neck and pulled me into a hug. We stood in the hallway for some time, each muttering sentiments of bewilderment, shock, and amazement. There was no big jump up and down moment; immediately, caution filled us. Everything felt calculated and methodical. Now it was time to get the plan together. We sat in the living room, my feet on Matt's lap and we got our plan together.

"I can't wait to tell everyone. I am too scared. I am going to need the family if it all goes wrong again."

Matt nodded quietly. "Agreed."

"And we need to call Natale."

"When do you start the blood thinner?"

"Not yet. In a couple weeks. I have to buy some."

"I will pick some up."

I glanced at him, as he was not reading the Sears flyer in front of him, his eyes staring through it. He is in full-protection mode already. This could be a long pregnancy.

In two days, we were going for dinner at Jane and Gus's house. It was a bitterly cold February day. As Matt pulled the car to a stop, I took a breath. Their beautiful stately home looked cozy and welcoming. Its large, white, wrap-around porch, and the smell from the wood fire, welcomed us in. I love their home and always feel as if we fully belong there. I didn't work up the courage until after dinner to say the sentence that was the constant thought in my mind;

"I am pregnant."

Before I knew what hit me, Jane's arms were wrapped around my neck as she sobbed. Pure relief and fear and grief and joy poured out of her. And me. And Gus. And Matt. We held each other and sobbed.

It was a long pregnancy. We knew from the start that anxiety would plague us. We did everything we could to manage it all in a calculated and disciplined fashion. I asked Dr. Natale to give me the warning signs and symptoms that would warrant me going into hospital immediately. He gave me a list, including seeing flashing lights, persistent headache, and upper-right-quadrant pain, amongst others. I placed the list on the fridge, and each and every day, I used that list to keep my mind and my anxiety steady. I also called on Kathy, and used EMDR therapy anytime I felt I needed to.

The first trimester was much the same as Ava's, only with less malaise. With my anxiety being increased, my nausea started early, and I was soon back to the same routine that I was in before of extra sleep and lots of rest. The biggest difference this time was the fact that I simply did not care who or what I affected. I was merciless with my self-care, to such a point that I knew that working would not last long. Around 9 weeks pregnant, I remember getting up one morning and seeing a very distinct baby bump.

"Matt! Come look at this," I said with a laugh to my voice.

"What?" he asked, as he rounded the corner while munching a piece of toast.

"Look!" I pointed to my sideways belly. "Am I supposed to be able to go to work looking like this?"

Looking down, it could be seen quite clearly: a baby bump. As if my coworkers were not keyed in enough to wonder what our family plans were.

"May I suggest sweatshirts?"

"To work?"

"Rub your eyes a lot and say you are feeling poorly?"

That was his suggestion? Feign sick and dress like a slob? This was not going to work. I knew I would have to tell them before it was more than apparent, for honesty's sake. They had been very supportive of us and our journey. I knew they would want to share in this too.

I managed to hold out to 11 weeks. Eleven weeks of sweatshirts and baggy clothes. Of folding down my pants, and wondering when someone would ask about the crackers on my desk. They responded with the compassionate, loving outpouring I had become very grateful for.

I worked until 18 weeks, at which point, my medical appointment frequency and self-care needed to improve. To keep my stress on the level, and to complete all the frequent medical appointments, giving myself fully to my position was impossible. The day I left the office, I knew I was not ever going to be returning. I knew it was over. My contract would not be renewed after this second departure, and I could tell from the air of politics that my time was done. I packed my carton and Matthew came to pick me up. I was relieved and sad, but mostly resolute. I felt like I was able to give a proper goodbye to the place I never did after Ava, and that felt good.

Being off work, self-care became easier. I rested when I needed to, and abided by my doctor's rules. And rules there were! So many, many rules. I cannot express the amount that Dr. Natale ruled my life. I am not allowed to lift over 20 pounds. Feet must be up three hours per day. Attend the hospital at a moment's notice. I must slow down, but not become inactive. I cannot babysit on my own for an extended period. I am to meditate and exercise every day. And above all, I must manage my stress levels. Notice how many things contradict each other? Yeah, I did too.

There were times when the restrictions were a scapegoat. When I knew something would not be good for me, and his voice in the back of my head would keep me in line. There were also times when breaking them just a little felt fantastic as well. With each passing week, the level of control that the hospital was having seeped in a bit more.

Every medical appointment lasted for hours. The appointments were at the hospital, and at a moment's notice, my doctor could be pulled away. It often meant grueling, long stretches of waiting to be seen, hours sitting in a small room, shifting and hoping you are not in the bathroom when your name is called. I geared up for hospital days, and would allow myself downtime after them.

We remained committed to doing things differently with this baby. We never had a nickname for Ava, so fairly early in the pregnancy, we set to finding a nickname for the wee one. One morning, while puttering around the kitchen, I asked Matthew,

"What comes after Alpha?"

"What do you mean?"

"The first time you do a test, it is called the Alpha test, right? Well, what is the second test called?"

"Beta."

Our eyes met and we chuckled. Beta. Our second try at this experiment called life. Beta somehow stuck, much to the chagrin of all of my family members. They were terrified that this nickname would continue in real life, but it never would. Beta was an affectionate way for us to say, "let us try again."

Shortly after I stopped work, we were scheduled for our anatomy scan. I was no stranger to ultrasounds. I had already had three. It was always an anxiety inducing moment when the wand would be placed on my belly and I would be waiting to hear them say, "I just need to get the doctor." However, we had yet to hear that.

Matthew came with me to the anatomy scan with the purpose that we would find out the baby's health and gender together. They told me the usual routine; drink an incredible amount of water and hold it before your appointment. This instruction is never necessary for me because of how I carry my babies. Inevitably, I end up too full and they make me relieve myself "partly" because my bladder is an obstruction to the procedure. This time, I drank one full glass of water and called it even, hoping that it would be enough. Surely it was.

Each ultrasound I had been through was the same. I was welcomed back. They completed the medical side of the appointment and then Matthew was welcomed back to see the baby. Anatomy scans can take longer. However, we were anticipating him waiting for half an hour before being called back to join me.

Not two hours.

Two hours he sat, terrified that something was wrong. Two hours where he was terrified to leave the room for fear that they would come for him and he wasn't there. Two hours wondering what was happening with his wife and child. Two hours that I lay on a table, holding my pee with a woman completing an ultrasound, who would not even tell me if the baby was okay. I was shaking. I begged her to simply show me that the baby was alive and I was told,

"I am not permitted. You must wait to talk to your doctor."

By the time she released me to go and wait for my doctor, I was in tears. Luckily, Matthew and I were able to regroup before going in to see Dr. Natale. When he came in to see us, I saw his eyes soften immediately. We were not quite halfway through our journey together, and he had yet to see me break down from sheer stress. I saw his demeanor adjust immediately.

"Well, Melissa. You have a healthy baby."

Matt and I clutched hands and breathed a sigh of relief. He updated us on all of the placenta functioning, and turned the screen towards us so we could see our baby. He then explained that the reason the scan took so much longer was because he was having the placental functioning examined. With each sentence, he said we sunk back in our chairs and breathed deeply. Before I knew it, he was beginning to wrap up the appointment.

"Dr. Natale. Were you able to see the gender?" I asked.

A smirk went across his face. He sat back in his chair and he smiled broadly at us. "Well, are you sure you want to know? Because once you know..."

"Yes. I need to bond. I really want to know."

As I spoke, Matt nodded along; we were ready to know.

"Well, let me just check. The other room has a better computer." He stood up with a spring to his step and left us waiting.

"Are you sure you want to know?" I asked Matt.

"Yes. Absolutely."

Matt isn't the guessing kind. I knew better than to ask. I thought it was a boy. In my family, each person has a girl followed by a boy. Ava was our girl and this would be our boy. I needed to know so I could bond with a son. A son would be completely different and everything in this pregnancy felt different. So it must be a boy.

Dr. Natale returned to the room, looking like a cat with the cream. His smile was sly as he slid into his chair. Looking at us both he said,

"XX."

"Really?" I exclaimed.

"Pardon?" Matt said. I looked at Matt and saw his confusion.

"XX!" I said. I could feel the tears burning my eyes and my throat catch.

Matt did not know what he meant.

"It is a girl," I squeaked.

"A girl?" Matt's entire face lit up as I broke down in tears.

Dr. Natale was confused by my reaction. "Is this a good thing?"

"Yes! Oh yes! A girl!"

He shook Matthew's hand and left us to collect ourselves. A girl. We would be having a sister for Ava.

Managing stress from 26 weeks out became incredibly difficult. With each passing week, we drew closer and closer to the 34-week mark. My doctor was fairly clear with me that HELLP would not present before its original presentation, which would mean that we would most likely not have HELLP if we were to get it until after 34+6. And the days began to click closer and closer.

We kept our eyes on the prize and continued our mantra, one appointment at a time. As the appointments went up to weekly, I could feel my anxiety rise. As did my blood pressure. Each appointment was always the same; wait for a potentially long and painful amount of time to be called in for weighing and blood pressure. So much of whether this would be a HELLP pregnancy was based off of my blood pressure. The intensity of that moment of sitting in the chair for the test was excruciating. Week by week, it kept ticking up.

Then one day, I saw flashing lights as I sat in the chair. Flashing lights were one of the risk factors Dr. Natale had so urgently warned me to watch for. Upon coming into the examination room, he did not mince words.

"Your BP is high. Why?"

I was dumbfounded. I did not know how to answer him. I felt completely taken aback and so sad, I could cry and vomit all at once.

"I do not know," I managed to squeak out.

I saw him sit back on his heels and stare at me. "Let's take a look at your baby." He wheeled in the portable ultrasound and put the wand to my belly. There she was, kicking and happy, our wee Beta baby.

"I need you to go downstairs to triage for monitoring," he said, his tone soft and assertive. "We need to monitor your blood pressure and see what is happening. If it comes down, then you can go home. But we need to keep an eye on it..."

As he spoke, the world began to spin. This is it. Here it starts again. Thirty weeks pregnant and here we go again. I began to shake all over as fury filled my body. Not again! This will not happen again. Of course, I was alone at the hospital, so they put me into a wheelchair and wheeled me down to triage, alone. I texted quickly to Matt, who was out of town, to let him know what was happening. Alone and in chaos. I wanted to cry.

No. Stay angry. I willed myself. I am going home today. This ends now.

They set me up in a triage room and a nurse met me with a warm smile.

"Alright, my dear, let us get you hooked up to the monitoring here," she said as she placed a band on my stomach. Immediately, I could hear Beta's heartbeat fill the room. I laid back and put my head on the bed.

"When was the last time you have eaten?" she asked softly.

"What time is it now?"

"2 p.m."

I had last eaten breakfast. My appointment was for 10 a.m., and I had been in hospital the entire time.

"Breakfast."

"Oh, you must be famished. Let me bring you a few nibbles. And you can sit back and relax."

Her tone and demeanor told me she knew the truth. She knew about Ava. She had read the chart and was told to handle with care. Normally, I would find this moment patronizing and I'd have been frustrated by it, but I found myself leaning into it for comfort.

Rubbing my belly, I said, "Alright, Beta. This wasn't the plan for today. Let's get this pressure down so we can go home and rest, together." I felt her kick in assurance and I curled slightly onto my side and wrapped my arms around my belly.

Bonding is hard. I found myself holding back a piece of my heart from her. Lying on this bed, alone with her, my blood pressure precariously high, and suddenly, I am faced with bonding or else. I need to use our bond to drive my blood pressure down. I can will this. Closing my eyes, I began to tap my legs as EMDR therapy taught me to. Breathing deeply and slowly, I force myself to calm. I can feel my phone buzzing against my leg and I ignore it. I have to do this. I have to let her in. Leaning into the sound of her heartbeat, I allowed myself to just let her in.

I heard the door open and I looked up to see the nurse returning to my room. She set down ginger ale and butter cookies on the side table.

"I will take your first blood pressure reading in a few minutes, my dear. Sit and rest."

I nodded in return and closed my eyes once more.

"Come on, Beta. We can do this. You and me, kid. Talk to me, Beta. Just let me know. Tell Mama and I will figure it out."

It would be another 10 minutes of quiet time and a small snack, but I began to feel a bit more myself. The nurse came in and took my blood pressure.

"Well, that is nearly saintly," she said with a smile.

"Is it coming down?"

She smiled and nodded in return, and left once more to return in another ten minutes.

Matthew was texting furiously that he was coming to the hospital to be with me. I assured him it was not necessary, that I was getting my pressures down, and I would be home that night. After a few more series' of pressure checks, Dr. Natale returned to the room.

"You seem to have this in hand," he said with a smirk. "But I want you to return in the morning. And the morning after that for a non-stress test and blood pressure monitoring." It was past 5 p.m., and I was simply exhausted, famished, and begging for home. I promised to do whatever is necessary just to go home and try again tomorrow. He saw the drawn resolve behind my eyes and said it was safe for me to go home.

I fairly bolted for the door. The second I arrived home, I called Kathy.

"I blew a high number with my blood pressure. It was all a head game. As soon as I calmed and listened to the baby, my BP came right down. We have to get this in hand."

Together, we talked about measures to get me through the next two days of appointments. Each time, Beta and I passed with flying colors. My BP was higher than normal, but controlled, and she was happy and kicking away.

The very next day, I went in to see Kathy once more, this time with my home blood pressure cuff in hand.

"It is a cycle. They are watching my blood pressure so closely, it is making me nervous, and then my blood pressure goes up. So they watch me closer, which makes me more nervous... This is insanity!"

"The doctors must be scared, too," Kathy responded. "They want to get her here safely too. Blood pressure is one of the only ways to figure out if anything is going wrong."

"So what do we do now? How do I keep myself steady in the midst of this medical... madness?"

Kathy hatched a plan, using EMDR to our advantage to deal with the trauma trigger of the pressure cuff. Using a hand temperature probe, the blood pressure cuff, and EMDR simultaneously, we watched my body's reactions to completing the session. Over the course of the hour, we watched my blood pressure fall slowly to its real normal, along with the warming of my hands from the coldness of trauma. Together, we went back over and over until I could feel the trigger diminish and new neural pathways form.

At the end of the two sessions, I knew what I had to do. Each and every time I had my blood pressure checked, I would tap my knees in the same manner we did in the EMDR sessions. If items came up that needed to be processed, I was to stop. However, if not, I was tasked with breathing into it and allowing myself to lean into the calm of the EMDR.

The next appointment was two days later that week and I practiced extensively at home. At least twice a day, I checked my blood pressure and would go through the same routine of tapping and breathing during the tests. I marched back into the hospital, head held high, ready to try again.

And it worked.

Dr. Natale noticed right away at the next appointment.

"It would appear as though your blood pressure is normal."

"Yes. I used EMDR therapy. I will continue to."

"Therapy?" He sat back in his chair, putting his hands behind his head. I know him well enough; he does that when he is figuring something out, curious and contemplating the angles.

"Yes," I said, my gaze meeting his.

He nodded in agreement.

"So as we have discussed prior, I went from having a difference in my platelets, to having HELLP syndrome in five days with Ava. I would like to have my platelet levels monitored weekly by blood draws."

"At that frequency, you could become anemic. I have other methods of monitoring the start of HELLP, including ultrasound."

"I agree. However, I do not trust it. I need to know the platelet numbers to feel this is in hand."

"I am concerned you would become fixated on the numbers."

"I already am. We are in the end of this now, so now is the time to know the numbers and ready ourselves."

"Weekly blood draws and ultrasounds to monitor blood flow, as well as appointments starting next week then," Dr. Natale pronounced.

I nodded in agreement. Having the upper hand, I knew what I needed to do.

One of the greatest moments of joy in my second pregnancy was given to me by my dear friend, Jane. Everyone wanted her here safely for us and for themselves, and they were eager to help. So eager, in fact, that I had to place my sister Kath as a liaison between myself and the well-wishers to allow me to focus. There is something so acutely anxiety-provoking in being asked continually how you are. Kath acted quickly to help send mass e-mails and to provide me well needed distance from those that meant well but could do me harm. Those that were close, I wanted nearby, and I could feel their palpable and genuine excitement and love for us. The very thought of a baby shower was anxiety inducing. Ava had died a few short days after her shower and I did not want the innocence and naivety that came with a shower. Jane approached me and offered to throw me a High Tea.

"Whoever you want. Just a ladies High Tea. Punch and champagne, finger foods, no presents, no games... What do you think?"

I instantly adored the idea, having all those people that support and love me in one space. It was a way to bring everyone together, nearing the end of my pregnancy and rallying everyone around. A way of including them and showing them how much I appreciated them.

On a muggy day in July, we gathered on Jane's sweeping front verandah for tea. There were paper lanterns and Gerber daisies hung in the hot shade with beautiful sparkling table settings, as 15 of my closest women gathered around to celebrate Beta and I, and to celebrate the courage and the will it took, to buoy me up and hold me longer. And it worked.

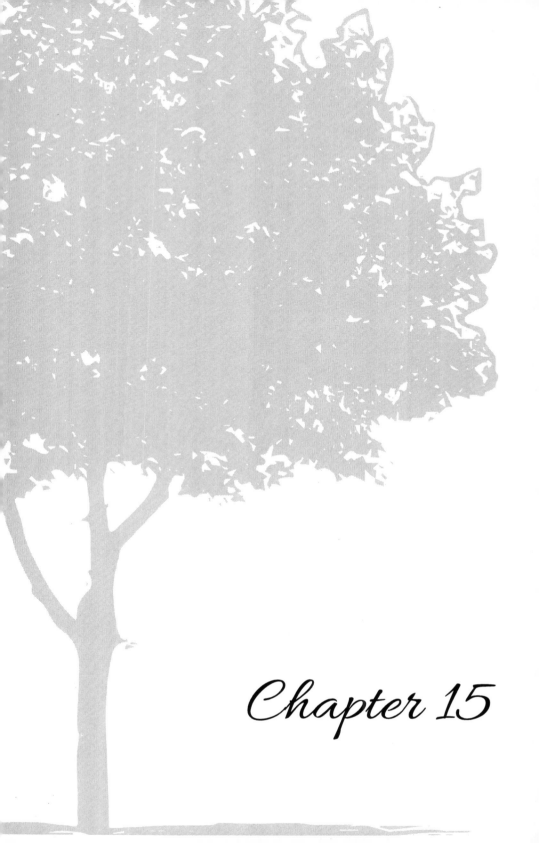

Chapter 15

She is Here!

Her birthday came with speed. One day, it was a star-marked day on the calendar, and the next moment, I was obsessively packing and repacking our bag the night before the big day. We were scheduled for an 8 a.m. C-section, which meant we were to be in the hospital, checked in by 6 a.m., and we live over half an hour away. The wake-up call for one of the most important days of our lives would be 4:45 a.m., and it loomed over our day before.

Both of us not knowing what you are supposed to do with yourself the night before decided that we needed something big, distracting, and in-your-face funny. Clearly, this called for *Austin Powers*. We lay in bed together, my head on his chest and his hand on my belly, as we watched every moment, attempting to get into the humor of it all. I felt proud that we were not pacing and obsessing like we wanted to at heart; our laughter and love filled the room, and I enjoyed the fact I felt safe, not knowing when that feeling would come again.

Poor Matthew barely slept a wink that night. I felt him leave bed sometime around 12:30 a.m. to go sleep on the couch. I didn't follow him, knowing that there was little I could do or say to ease his mind. I had the same concerns, yet I slept. Lying in bed, I felt a finality wash over me. I had no control over the next day. I had no control over what would or wouldn't happen. I was ready. I was oddly calm and resting well. The next morning, I awoke with excitement. Today was her day. Our day. No matter what, it would be answered today. I could see the fear in Matt's eyes. I know that fear, but did not share it. I put my hands on my belly. I was ready.

Check in for our C-section was routine. The hardest moment was changing out of my clothes and into the hospital gown. I remember doing this with Ava and the extreme agony I was in at the time.

"Breathe, Melissa. Breathe." My hands shook with fear as I pulled the gown over my belly. "Be present. Be present."

Routine questions, routine procedures and blood draws, and the first hour flew by. My parents arrived, as did our midwife, Laura. Their excitement was palpable. It filled the room and made me even calmer and more assured. All of the sudden, our nurse, Mariam, walked in. Mariam, who spent the night with us when Ava died. She was an ultimate comfort to Matthew. I had mentioned her name to our doctor, hoping that we would be able to involve her in Lillian's birth. She did not know we were her patients that day. She was simply told she would be participating in a C-section. When she came around the corner and she saw Matt and I, she undid at the seams. The entire group was together again, and somehow... Ava was there. I basked in this moment; all the work came down to this—and Ava was there. Somehow, it felt like she was present and participating fully in this moment. My heart swelled, and I thought for just a moment, maybe, it would be okay.

Of course, then the anesthesia came in to consult and despite all the meetings, my advocating, and the hospital advocating for us, they denied us having Matthew present for the spinal. They would allow Laura and stated that Matthew could stand at the door, looking in. A mere three feet away, but not present. With little choice, I accepted it. The time for fighting was over. Now it was time to survive. I would show them dignity.

Sitting on the operating table with Katie in front of me, I begged her to tell me the most inappropriate story she knew. Her face laughed at the request, but I could see the stress in her eyes. I clung to her, knowing that we could do this, together. Over her shoulder, Matthew was standing at the window of the door, his face staring intently at mine. His blue eyes were buried into mine, his fierceness was palpable and reached across the feet we were separated. They asked me to round my shoulders and I told Katie to talk louder and, preferably, with more emphatic swear words. She gladly obliged. As they put in the spinal, I prepared myself for the worst. Pain? Nausea? Perhaps a medical crash that would result in intubation?

"There you go, Melissa. That is the worst part."

What was the worst part? Nothing happened yet!

Apparently the spinal went in and I didn't even notice. I kept waiting for the world to stop spinning and it did not. Would this time be different?

They laid me down on the table, and I could feel 20 sets of hands on me at once. Trauma triggers ran through my body. Too many hands; it felt chaotic. I asked for Katie to tell me what was happening. Her face was in mine, explaining who everyone was and what they were doing, when I looked up and saw my doctor working on cleaning my stomach. I was immediately distracted, knowing that my doctor being in the room meant that he was in charge, and not anaesthesia. Instantly relieved, I said in a quiet voice,

"Dr. Natale, can I have Matthew now?" My voice shook with fear. Dr. Natale looked around and said, "Where is Matthew? Wasn't he supposed to be here?" There was an edge to his voice and his face disappeared as the curtain was raised between us.

"Hey, you." Matthew's soft tone filled my ears and I felt myself relax into his presence.

"How you doing?"

"Nauseous. Shaky." I felt like I could shake off the table at any moment, my fear raging so loud, it rang in my ears. Matthew came close to me and put his face in mine; his eyes were no longer scared but strong. I reassured him that I was okay, our chatter quiet and calm. He stroked the bridge of my nose and held my hand, all the while making me laugh with inside jokes. Katie was close. I could hear her banter softly. All of the sudden, I felt the doctor reach into my stomach. An overwhelming sense of nausea waved over me, as his hand felt like it was inside my stomach and my entire body was trapped. I could not move away. It was a horrid, awful feeling, and I could barely breathe. Gripped with terror, I gasped,

"Oh, God, I am going to be sick!"

"No, you won't." Dr. Natale's voice was firm, as it felt like he was reaching up to my throat. Every sensation made my body scream in terror. It felt wrong and completely chaotic. I gasped for breath, panting.

"Oh God, Matt. Oh God, Matt."

Matt's eyes were worried and trained on mine.

"Breathe. Breathe."

He grabbed my hand firmly and came so close, I swear our noses touched.

My eyes watering from chaos and fear, I gripped him firmly and begged for the courage to bear it one moment longer.

And then I heard her.

A sputter.

A screech.

A full belly cry.

Could that be?

I stared up at the ceiling, my eyes groping at the top of the curtain for her. Searching.

"Look up, Melissa, here she is!"

Lillian!

Epilogue

Look at them there.

Father and daughter.

He is trying to feed Lillian some pepper from the picnic supper I had packed. Her eager 7-month-old self, one tooth and all the determination in the world is not enough to get that red slice in her mouth fast enough. I see panic in his eyes as she gums off a large piece and she is going for the swallow. I reach across the picnic table and swipe it out of her mouth, break it apart, and hand-feed it slowly to her.

She kicks her legs and squawks in protest. His panic diminishes. I can see his heartrate slow from here.

And the sun feels good.

I tilt my head back to put the sun in my face, try to breathe, and be present. It is hard, though.

"Her tree has really grown." Matt's observance interrupts my quiet moment.

I glance over at her tree and see, somehow, it has grown substantially since we planted it, just two years ago. It makes me smile that it is healthy and growing, but it stings. She should be two and growing, and I shouldn't be sitting here; rather, I should be chasing her on the monkey bars over there. The realization of the sticky sister kisses that Lillian is missing stings my eyes and I am glad for my sunglasses; he would feel bad if he saw his that comment tripped me down the grief wormhole.

"Yes," I said as I shook my head to clear the grief, "it really has."

I stare down at my belly. Still deflating, 7 months later. These two girls have taken their toll. It is unsettling to find yourself in a body and place in life you never thought you would ever have. Multi-layered, I never thought I would actually bring her here alive. Lillian, that is. I had picked a spot beside Ava's tree for Lillian's as well.

How sick is that? Picking out the memorial for the child you have yet to birth. These are the things we tell ourselves to survive.

I don't think Matt and I have moved from survival mode. Like the panic of the pepper in her mouth, there is a part of us that is waiting for the next crisis. Part of me has a fear that is so gripping and just beneath the surface, forever changing who I am.

I am not the parent I thought I would be. When she was 2-months-old, we took Lillian for her vaccinations and that night, when I put her to bed, she felt hot. Adrenaline rushed through my body and I managed to croak out to Matthew for him to help strip her naked, do a cool bath and get the fever medicine. An eternity later, my world was moving in slow motion, swallowing bile down my throat, heart racing as I took her temperature again and again; it finally began to lower. I sat on the floor with her in my arms and inconsolably rocked her with gigantic tears streaming down my face. She was perfectly fine. I, however, was not. It took hours for me to stop shaking from that first 38.3 degree fever. Earning my dues as a Mama was far harder than I ever could have imagined. All of this was with a freight train of grief and PTSD carried on my back.

We have had the same learning curves as any "new" parents, however, with a new burden of fear and grief interlaced into every experience. Mom and baby groups where they ask upon arrival:

"How many kids do you have?"

And I gulp hard and consider my options. Do I want to air all my business to these strangers? If I say two, but my first was stillborn, the room falls quiet and I can see them physically pull away and somehow, out of somewhere, a freak label comes out and is stamped onto my forehead. I will spend the rest of the time with the other Moms skirting my eye contact and keeping their children to their knee. But I am gripped with guilt each and every time I deny her existence to save face. I apologize to her under my breath time and time again, when I state "I only have one." It is an impossible choice, each moment with a different answer. There are times where I say her name simply because I need to hear it, and times where I tell the flat-out truth to a complete strangers, also as a way to shock and awe them into realizing life isn't all rainbows and kittens.

Mothering is now plagued with questions I never thought I would have to answer. How do I explain Ava to Lillian in a way that does not damage or place expectation on her? So many people assumed that, as soon as we had a second daughter, we had "replaced" Ava. That notion diminishes both girls; neither is replaceable and they hold equal value and sacred space in our family. Not to mention, it is entirely crass and as shallow as a saucer of milk. You can replace goldfish, not children. Our wee family has a complication to it that sets it aside from the norm in so many ways. Yet, all we are is a "normal" family attempting to figure out this thing called life together. We are trying to figure out colic and growth spurts, diaper ointments and teething. All those delicious baby things we craved and yearned for, for so, so long.

Sometimes, I wonder how this will all be from Lillian's perspective. The big sister that is lost, her Mama's large snaking scar, our friends and loss families with everyone missing a sibling, her parent's tears, the tree. Our Ava's tree, which we decorate every Christmas Eve so she can hear the bells ring for her in Heaven. Where we picnic with family and friends, all in the shade of her boughs. Our Lillian will grow in the shade of her big sister Ava's tree and she will outgrow, outrun, and outlive its life.

Seeing the two of them, on our picnic blanket in the spring sun, him tossing her gently in the air and hearing her squeals of delight, all framed against the background of her tree, somehow, it feels complete. As complete as incomplete can get and somehow, that is enough.

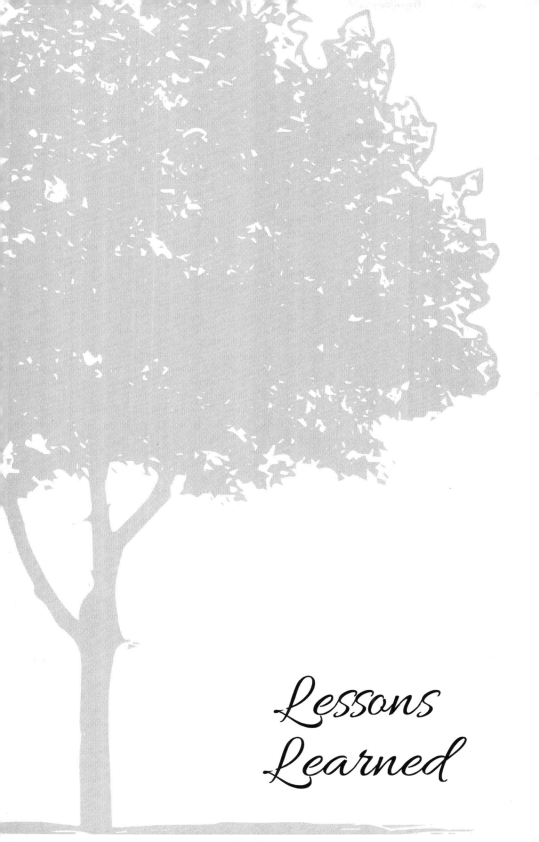

Lessons
Learned

Navigating a Pregnancy After Loss

My survival strategy to surviving a high-risk pregnancy or a pregnancy after loss.

1) Getting your team together: a) medical, b) emotional, and c) self-care.

The importance of getting a team together cannot be understated in navigating a pregnancy after loss. It takes a village to raise a child as well as to birth one. In high-risk pregnancies, this is especially true, as often times, there are many different medical professionals consulting on one "file". "Getting your team together" is about accessing your NEEDS for this pregnancy. Do you NEED to have certain medical tests prior to becoming pregnant? Access your medical needs in tandem to your emotional needs. Do you NEED to hear the baby's heartbeat at each medical visit? Do you NEED bloodwork or certain testing regularily to help you keep your anxiety in check? Do you NEED trauma counselling to help you manage the stress and anxiety?

Ask yourself, together as a couple, what your needs are and communicate them to your team. It is also advantageous to have a leader to your medical team, typically whoever is in charge of your medical care. Be sure to choose a team leader that is comfortable in dealing with whoever else is part of this process (i.e., Midwives, family members, chiropractor, psychotherapist, counsellor). Do your homework, sign release forms, and allow all members to talk to one another as you need. That way, everyone is on the same page together. Most importantly of all, once you have your team, trust them.

2) Stress management is self-care

It will not be possible for you to be relaxed in this pregnancy. What is most important is that you manage your stress level. For your child's sake and for your sanity and health, being on top of and actively managing stress is imparative. Managing stress does not mean sitting at a spa and telling yourself you are fine. Managing stress means doing those things that help you feel less stressed. It does not have to be what others think will work; instead, it has to be what works for you. Think of your grief. In the darkest moments, what helped? What helped you pick yourself off the kitchen floor from the sheer agony of screaming for your child? Was it a phone call to a friend? Was it slapstick humour or walking the dog? Stress management in a pregnancy after loss is self-care. They are one in the same. Take a moment and ask yourself what you need; do you need to call your midwife, hear the baby's heartbeat, and go have lunch with a friend? Do it.

I also encourage taking this pregnancy one moment at a time. You have survived grieving and living; you can survive this too.

3) You are your baby's advocate

If we blame ourselves when our baby dies, then we have to allow ourselves to advocate for our child that is living. A scary concept but the reality is, there is no mother of a child that dies that has not asked themselves what they did wrong and how they could have prevented it. You are not accountable when your baby dies. It is not your fault. Allow yourself to advocate for their life. Do not be afraid to be "that" woman who is constantly at the triage, saying she has not felt the baby move. Do not be afraid to rock the boat and make your team work for you. Your team wants this for you. They would not be beside you if they didn't, so push! Ask! Question! You are the advocate, so you know best. Dig deep inside yourself and LISTEN.

Do whatever you need to do to hear your baby. Talk to your baby, communicate what is happening and why. This communication bond is sacred, and it will serve you to be able to hear what is needed. Many women describe a need for quiet and calm, and giving yourself that will allow you to advocate even better because you will be able to hear your own voice, your mother's intuition, and the baby's soul speaking to you, through you.

I knew, for example, that my rainbow baby could not stand ultrasounds in the beginning. I knew they made her head hurt. I could feel how loud they felt to her. Ultrasounds were hard to avoid in my high-risk pregnancy, since I needed them to assure her safety. So I talked to my team about reducing them to a minimum and then I talked to her. I would tell her when they were coming, I would tell her what was happening and I felt she needed quiet for the day after, so we would do the ultrasound and I would be very quiet for the rest of the day. Calm, soothing music. Long baths with running water. Hushed tones. In time, I knew the ultrasounds were not as bad for her and I know it helped her a great deal in dealing with them. Listen; if your gut says it, you are right.

4) People management

People management is important. Well-meaning people intrude. Not-well-meaning people are worse. They can mess with your head, ask all sorts of questions, and rock you off your very slippery and fragile equilibrium for their own gain, with little idea of the damage they have done. I assigned a People Manager in my team. This is the person that communicated with everyone about the 5000 questions I was asked on a daily basis. This is the person who would field questions and that I could say, call so-and-so; they will tell you all about it. This is also useful for when the baby comes home and you need some space and quiet, and all the people in your life are already used to asking your sister, so they go to her to ask when they can come by or if they can drop off food.

Part of people management is also cleaning your house and recognizing who is not healthy for you. Ask yourself what this person contributes and what role you want them to play. In that lies your answer of how involved you should make them. People management is all about your choice.

5) Set milestones, rewards, and celebrate this life as the unique thing it is

You will never get to be pregnant with this baby again. You will never get these moments again. Remember wishing for one more moment? Well, this is your moment with this person. Think ahead and set yourself milestones and celebrate them. Is it "viability" that matters to you? Perhaps finding out the gender ahead of time? Create memories with this baby unique to him or her. This child does not live in the shadow nor replaces his or her sibling. Celebrate! My firstborn daughter died at 34+6, so once a week, after I went out for poutine. It was my reward. Little milestones, big milestones. All of them; mark them.

6) Allow yourself to bond

This was the hardest part of a pregnancy after loss for me. Allowing myself to feel this baby and love this baby, knowing, as I do, that it all can slip through my fingers. The reality is, to advocate for and celebrate this baby, you must allow yourself to bond. This is your chance, your moment to love this little person; come what may, this is it. What does this wee one like? Dislike? Write letters and journals to remember it all along the way.

7) Allow yourself to grieve

Grief ignored is grief waiting for you. Your grief process will continue, even though you are pregnant. I say process because that is what it is, a process that continues day by day. Do what you need to grieve. You are not hurting this baby by grieving; in fact, you are taking care of yourself. Pent up grief places pressure on your heart and soul and muddles the communication and connection you can have with your growing babe. Allow the grief to flow, and tell this baby about his or her sibling. Allow that space and continue your grief rituals.

8) Bringing the baby home

Isn't this the big goal? To bring a living, breathing baby home. Guess who will complicate it? People. "You don't have the nursery set up? You wanted to breastfeed for so long, so how could you not now? Do you have a birth plan? Make a plan! Make a plan!"

Some couples need the nursery set up. I needed a nursery to grieve in. In case my second born did not survive, I needed a room that was hers to grieve her in. Some people cannot FATHOM setting up a crib. There is no right answer to any of these issues. Rather, what is important is doing what works for you. Bringing your baby home will be in the pinnacle of your team working together. It is when your team will be the most taxed and you will need them the most. Rely on them and allow yourself the permission to do whatever you need to for your sanity.

How to Support the Bereaved

Things to Not Do or Say

(written by Melissa Krawecki and Carol Peat)

1) When my sister, mother, best friend died...

No two losses are alike and this statement changes the conversation to be about your grief and not supporting the person who is grieving.

2) I cannot imagine what you are going through.

I already feel like a freak of nature. I walk through the world, knowing that what happened to my family is rare and that most everyone else gets to have what I do not. Stating that you cannot imagine what I am going through makes me even more the freak than I already am. It also states pity, that my life is so terrible that you, from your dignified and gracely state, could not imagine the depravity of my life.

3) Let me know if there is anything I can do.

I have no idea what I want. This statement places pressure on the newly bereaved to have to search for something for you to do to comfort me. This statement is empty and shallow. There are better ways to offer support.

4) I could not do what you are doing. You are so strong.

I am not strong, I am polite. I am only doing what I have to because I have no other choice. I am standing here "strong" in front of you but I have my best face on, and you have not seen my pain.

5) I will bring your dinner tomorrow night.

Please do not bring me another lasagne; my freezer was stacked full of lasagnes for months on end. I could not eat while grieving in the early days, and food was often sent home with other people. I did not need food. I needed other help much more.

6) Happy 4th of July / Christmas / Hanukkah / Thanksgiving.

Nothing is "happy" after a child dies. I spent years dreaming of her first Christmas and instead, it was one of the worst days of my life. Holidays, even the smallest or seemingly insignificant ones, can be very difficult. Instead, try and find a way that you are remembering their child on that holiday, like mailing them an ornament or buying a gift for a child the same age and allowing them to see your actions in their child's name.

7) You will feel better eventually.

You do not know that.

8) What happened? (Tell me the story)

Having to retell a traumatic story is exhausting. And retelling the story for someone's amusement and entertainment is far worse. Each time a family retells their story, it is possible for them to relive their trauma with each word. Instead, be receptive to listening and if they wish to tell you, they will.

9) You are doing great.

In this moment, I APPEAR to be doing great. You are complimenting my ability to fake it in front of you. There are better compliments.

10) Your family is in my prayers.

Prayers are not for everyone.

Things to Do and Say

(Written by Melissa Krawecki and Carol Peat)

❧ Nothing at all. Hold the space. "I have no words."

❧ I hear you.

❧ You are not alone.

❧ Just breathe.

❧ If, and only if, the baby is physically present: "Let us focus on your baby as much as we can."

❧ Everything you would say for a living child. "He is beautiful! Look at his dark hair!"

❧ Pictures are important. May I take one for you?

❧ It is all normal. What you are feeling is normal.

❧ Let us spend time with the baby.

❧ Names are important.

❧ Would you like me to help you dress the baby?

❧ I have information about local funeral homes. Would you like me to help you with that process?

Tips to Help in the Moment

❧ Have a separate room apart from the live births.

❧ Do not rush the family out of the birthing area or hospital.

☞ The parents are in SHOCK. They do not know what appropriate behaviour is, and thus, highly persuadable. Do not abuse that.

☞ Talk about what they may be seeing: bleeding, tissue damage, etc.

☞ Parents will follow your lead easily; if you lead them to believe they should rush, they will. They will REGRET rushing.

☞ Respect confidentiality.

☞ Take cues from the family regarding management of the extended family.

☞ Tears are okay. Just never ask the patient or family to comfort you. Never apologize for crying.

☞ Respect the baby. Respect the body. Dignity. Always dignity.

Memorials

☞ Imagine, horridly for a moment, that you only get one moment EVER with your child for the rest of your life. Just one moment. This is their moment.

☞ Allow for the family to memorialize their child. Assist wherever you can.

☞ If invited to a formal memorial for the child at a later date, please consider going. You are an important tie to that child and the relationship you share will help in hard times.

Examples include: Footprints, handprints, locks of hair (multiple, if possible), pictures, bathing, dressing in multiple outfits, information about funeral homes.

Things to Help Trauma Victims

☞ Permission to touch. Always.

☞ Limit touch to whenever necessary. Each touch to a trauma victim is much stronger and could be bringing up very difficult memories. Respect that.

☞ Reduce stimuli–Lights, sounds; use a sound machine to block upsetting noises or the constant hum of the hospital.

☞ Talk through procedures prior to doing them. Talk throughout and summarize afterwards.

☞ Attempt to keep your trauma in check.

☞ Tears are okay, but never ask for the parents to comfort you.

☞ Listen to the patient.

☞ Make no assumptions in regards to family structure and supports. Consider advocates available and provide supports as seen fit. "Do you have anyone you would like to be here with you?" This includes hospital advocates.

☞ Provide social work contacts at an appropriate time.

☞ Encourage the traumatized to take back their power one thing at a time; be that self toileting or a face wash. Listen to the choices they are making for themselves and honour them.

Made in the USA
Charleston, SC
30 June 2016